PSYCHIC ANATOMY YOGA

ON THE FRONT LINE OF EVOLUTION

SUPPORTED BY OVER 600 TRADITIONAL AND SCIENTIFIC REFERENCES

BRETT A. ROGERS

Table of Contents

Preface   1

Part 1: Psychic Energy Exercises

Section 1: The Core Psychic Energy Exercises

Chapter 1: Introduction to Psychic Anatomy Yoga   11

Chapter 2: The Very Beginning   19
    Posture
        Sitting Posture
        Kneeling Stools
        Standing Posture
    Breath
        Chest and Abdominal Breathing
    Visualizations and Affirmations
        The Fundamental Affirmations
    Music
    Sacred Space
    Meditation
        Experiential Meditation
    General Techniques
    Warm-up Routine
    Preparation Exercises
        Pulsate Breathing Exercise
        Full Body Pulsate Breathing Exercise

Chapter 3: Introduction to Psychic Anatomy   49

Chapter 4: Your Aura   **51**
Chakra Exercise 1
Chakra Exercise 2
Auric Body Exercise 1 and 2
Aura Exercise
Yin-Yang

Chapter 5: Meridians   **61**
Vessel Descriptions (Extraordinary Vessels)
Meridian Descriptions
Vessel Exercise 1
Vessel Exercise 2
Meridian Exercise
Comments on Vessel and Meridian Exercises
Nadi Exercise
Sushuma Exercise
Meridian Mudra
Combining Aura and Meridian Exercises
Working with Pockets of Unhealthy Psychic Energies
Meditation and Grounding Comments

Chapter 6: Your Hara   **87**
Hara Exercise
Tan Tien Exercise
Sine Wave

Chapter 7: Core Star   **95**
Core Star Exercise

Chapter 8: Working with Pockets of Psychic Energies   **99**
Working with Pockets of Unhealthy Psychic Energies
Working with Pockets of Healthy Psychic Energies

Chapter 9: Final Comments   **103**

Section 2: Intermediate Psychic Energy Exercises

Chapter 10: Heaven and Earth Exercises   **109**
    Conducting/Embracing Heaven
    Conducting/Embracing Heaven Exercise
    Embracing/Conducting Earth
    Embracing/Conducting Earth Exercise
    Bridging Heaven and Earth
    Arm Movements that Compliment Heaven and Earth Exercises
    Final Comments

Chapter 11: Some Final Exercises   **121**
    General Alignment
    Turning Inwards
    Ascending/Descending
    Cycling
    General Routine
    General Routine with Asanas
    Final Comments

Chapter 12: Final Comments on Part 1   **133**

Part 2: Incorporating Asanas

Chapter 13: Introduction   **139**

Chapter 14: On the Physical Topics of Asanas   **143**
    Cardiovascular Exercise
    Neck and Upper-Mid Back
    Hands, Wrists and Forearms
    Feet, Ankles, Calves and Shins
    Resisting/Engaging
    Centering Your Spine
    Static Variations
    Bouncing, Tapping and Shaking
    Breathing
       A Bahda Exercise
    Flushing with Fresh Blood
    Final Comments

Chapter 15: From Seated Part 1   **155**

Chapter 16: From Hands and Knees   **159**
Details on Threading the Needle
Details on Head Charging
Details on Crow
Details on Child's Pose

Chapter 17: From Standing on Knees   **167**
Details on Half Swimmer and Mountain Climber

Chapter 18: From Forward Fold   **173**

Chapter 19: From Down Dog   **177**
Details on Plank
Details on Pigeon

Chapter 20: From Standing   **185**
Details on Moving into/out of Standing from/to Forward Fold
Details of Leaning Back (Back Bend)
Details on Balancing Asanas
Details on Eagle
Details on Tree

Chapter 21: From Straddled Standing   **197**
Details on Standing Lunge
Details on Warrior 2
Benefits of a Kneeling Stool/Support Blocks

Chapter 22: Inversions   **205**
Details on Plough and Shoulder Stand
Details on Heaven and Earth Exercises

Chapter 23: From Seated Part 2   **207**
Details on Hamstring Stretch
Details on Neck Stretches

Chapter 24: From Lying   **211**
Details on Corpse

Chapter 25: Psychic Anatomy Yoga Flows   **215**
    Morning Routine
    Heat Series/Sun Salutations
    Ending Your Practice
    Ending Your Day

Chapter 26: Final Comments   **223**

Appendices

Appendix A: Group Practice   **227**

Appendix B: Group Exercises   **231**

Appendix C: Becoming a Teacher   **237**

Appendix D: Healthy Diet Hints   **247**

Appendix E: Liquid and Fasting Type Cleanses   **261**

Appendix F: Improving Brain Health and Performance   **269**

Appendix G: The Eight Limbs of Psychic Anatomy Yoga   **281**

Appendix H: Making a Kneeling, Meditation T and Wrist/Ankle Support Blocks   **285**

About the Author   **291**

Other Books and DVDs by Brett A. Rogers   **293**

In Person and Online Events   **311**

PREFACE

Psychic Anatomy Yoga is a new form of Yoga, but if you look at the history of Yoga, it is more similar to ancient forms than modern ones. These ancient forms (ex. kundalini and tantra yogas) focus on cultivating and controlling different types of psychic energies, which they called sakti and prana[1]. Psychic Anatomy Yoga cultivates and controls psychic energies in the same and different ways. Its major difference is how it includes psychic anatomy more directly, as well as some other improvements as a result of my research into similar practices[2] from around the world and associated scientific studies.

You may have heard something about your psychic anatomy before. It is the parts of you that works with psychic energies. It includes your aura and its chakras and auric bodies, your meridians (also known as nadis), your hara and its tan tiens, as well as your core star. These parts of you are introduced in Section ?[3]. Many details concerning psychic anatomy can be found in historical records and practices from around the world. Some parts can also be found in more modern scientific studies along with psychic energies[4].

Your psychic anatomy interfaces with your physical body in many ways. This is the mind-body-spirit connection. As the health and performance of your psychic anatomy increases or decreases, your body reflects this. Psychic Anatomy Yoga enhances your physical health and performance with asanas as most form of yoga do, but it also helps to reduce the presence

---

[1] Table 1, in Chapter 1, is a list of over 25 different names for these energies from around the world.

[2] Ex. Qi-gong, Tai Chi and Energy Healing.

[3] See my book *The Psychic Anatomy Exercises* for a more detailed discussion or my book *The Psychic Energy Reality* for a scientific discussion.

[4] Many studies are discussed in *The Psychic Energy Reality* and *The Interface Between Psychic Energies and the Physical Body*.

of unhealthy psychic energies within your psychic anatomy, as well as help to empower healthier ones. Details are discussed in Section 1.

You may have heard that energy (aka. psychic energies) follows thought. A more precise way of saying this is that psychic energies are attracted, empowered and directed with focused attention/intention. Every emotion and thought you give attention to, attracts and empowers associated psychic energies within your psychic anatomy and/or projects them from you. A phenomenon many of us have experienced.

This phenomenon has many implications. When it comes to Psychic Anatomy Yoga, it is used to enhance the health and performance of your psychic anatomy and physical body. Many modalities do this, but only Psychic Anatomy Yoga[5] incorporates a full spectrum of psychic anatomy exercises to maximize benefits!

Aside from my extensive research into psychic anatomy, I have also gone to great lengths studying similar practices, such as energy healing modalities, qi-gong, yoga, self-help[6] and more. This has led me to incorporate and develop other great techniques, such as working with pockets of psychic energies, Heaven and Earth Exercises, General Alignments, Ascending/Descending and more; discussed in Section 1.

When combining these powerful psychic energy techniques with asanas, all benefits of asanas are enhanced and the ones involving psychic energies are greatly enhanced. The most significant psychic energy benefit is enhanced awareness of psychic energies, usually called Extra Sensory Perception or

---

[5] Psychic Anatomy Yoga is also taught in a more advanced way, as discussed in *Psychic Anatomy Exercises*. It can also be used as a form of energy healing, as discussed in *Psychic Anatomy Treatments*.

[6] Self-help is a powerful subject when it comes to working with psychic energies, because our psychology is greatly intertwined with our psychic energy abilities.

Clairvoyance. This awareness allows you to read between the lines of what another person says/writes or does not say/write. It also makes it easier to be become aware of your intuitive guidance. Both are big advantages for making decisions, especially in the decision-rich-busy life styles many of us lead.

Other benefits includes an enhanced ability to control psychic energies for healing and empowering purposes (discussed ??). General mental, emotional and physical health and performance is also enhanced. This is an example of the mind-body-spirit connection; discussed ??. Mental, emotional and physical health and performance can also be enhanced in more specific ways; discussed in ??.

The asanas also enhance the benefits of these psychic energy techniques in a few of ways. It is a beautiful symbiotic relationship. For example, asanas make it easier for psychic energies to flow threw the body, which makes it easier for psychic energies to do their thing. The asanas also engage the physical body and challenge it, which will help ground you from the expansive states of being associated with these exercises.

I've studied and practiced many psychic energy arts since 1995 and have put a lot of effort into making sure the teachings of Psychic Anatomy Yoga are as accurate and effective as possible[7]. My goal is to help people increase the health and performance of their psychic anatomy and physical body, making it easier for them to live to their fullest potential. It is my hope that you will use your enhanced state of being to continue evolving yourself, as well as contribute to our collective evolution. I believe this is the meaning of life[8].

---

[7] See my book *The Psychic Energy Reality* for an academic discussion with over 600 supporting references on the teachings of Psychic Anatomy Yoga.

[8] The meaning of life is discussed within *God's Journey/A Formula for Evolution.*

4

You've probably heard the saying that "we are all (of) one". The techniques in this book can help you experience this first hand. As you continue to practice, this reality, as well as others, will become more real (enlightenment), benefiting you and all of us :) :) .

"We are the ones we have been waiting for"

PART 1

PSYCHIC ENERGY EXERCISES

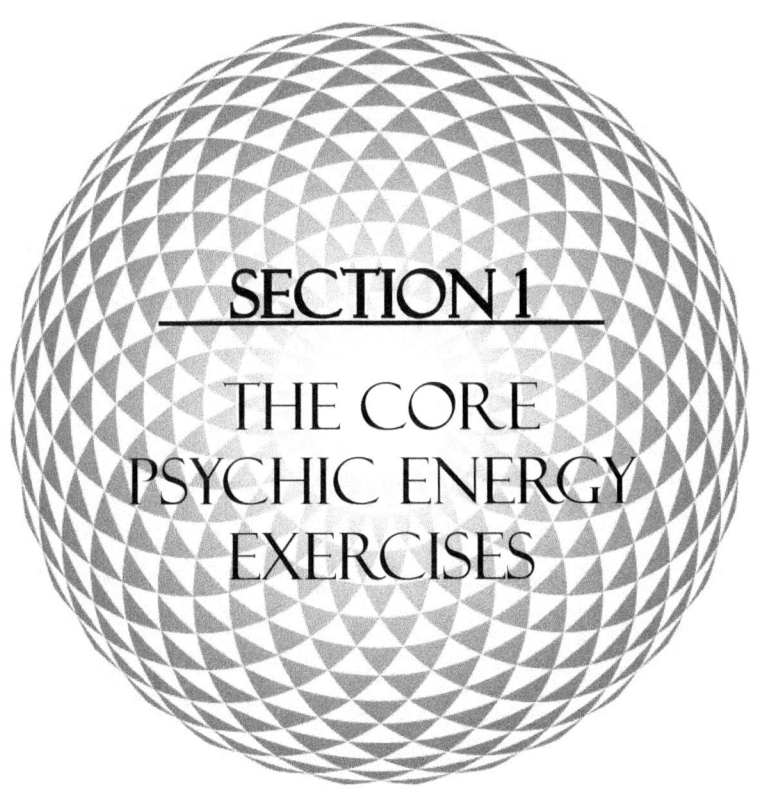

SECTION 1

THE CORE PSYCHIC ENERGY EXERCISES

CHAPTER 1
INTRODUCTION TO PSYCHIC ANATOMY YOGA

Psychic energies (PE) is the term I use to describe the energies associated with emotions, thoughts and spiritual experiences. They are the energies of our psyche/consciousness. You may be more familiar with the names other cultures have used, such as Chi/Qi in China, Ki in Japan, Ond in Poland, Mana in Hawaii, Gana in South America and others; see Table below. Common in yoga circles are the names Sakti and Prana.

Sakti is a more comprehensive word for these energies, while prana refers to more physically based sakti. You breathe prana into your lungs naturally and with practice, you can learn to do so more effectively. You can also learn to breath/absorb prana directly to your body, as well as your psychic anatomy; psychic anatomy discussed in Chapters 3-7. It is this breathing of prana that has led to the confusion that prana means "breath".

Although different cultures have different names and ideas about PE and psychic anatomy, there are many similarities as well. For example, how PE works, how to use them and some parts of our psychic anatomy. Modern research is starting to confirm and build upon these different ideas, which I am trying to contribute to[9].

The modern understanding on how PE work, which agrees with most traditions, is focused attention/intention attracts, projects and empowers PE associated with your attention/intention. This fundamental principle is the foundation of most practices

---

[9] See my books *The Psychic Energy Reality* and *The Interface Between Psychic Energies and the Physical Body* for in depth discussions.

involving PE, such as Psychic Anatomy Yoga.

Table: Cultural Names for Psychic Energies (PE)

Name for PE	Culture
Apu	Incan or Peru
Ankh	Ancient Egypt
Arunquiltha	Australian Aborigine
Gana	South America
Huaca	Peru/Bolivia
Ki	Japan
Mana	Polynesia
Mana	Hawii
Orenda	Iroquois Native Americans
Peneuma	Ancient Greece
Prana	India
Sakti	India
Qi/Chi	China
Ton	Dakota Native Americans
Walkan or ni	Lakota Native Americans
Spirit	Many Native American Tribes
Ashe	African
Ond	Poland
Orgone	North America/Europe
Tachyons	North America/Europe
Life Force	North America/Europe
Subtle Energy	North America/Europe
Spiritual Energies	North America/Europe
Healing Energies	North America/Europe
Ruach	Hebrew
Psyche	Greek
Spiritus	Latin
Astral Light	Kabbalists
Biological PK	Parapsychologist
Information collected from various authors	

Once PE merge with your body/psychic anatomy, the PE will influence you to bring your attention back to the things associated with them. This is essentially your unconscious/subconscious mind[10].

If you are mindful of how you focus your attention, you can cultivate healthy PE that will influence you towards healthy things. This will increase the health and performance of your mind-body-spirit (aka. physical body and psychic anatomy). Healthy PE enhance health and performance and unhealthy ones oppress health and performance.

The techniques of Psychic Anatomy Yoga empower healthy PE, making it easier for them to become apart of you. As you become more abundant in healthy PE, unhealthy PE that you took on in your past will start to be detoxified. The abundance healthy PE also makes it easier to resist taking on unhealthy PE from your environment and when interacting with other people in the moment.

This book will teach you to empower healthy PE in both general and specific ways. Chapters 3-7 will teach you about your psychic anatomy and some exercises for focusing specific types of healthy PE upon them. This helps to enhance their health and performance, which enhances your psychic abilities, as well as the health and performance of your mind, emotions and physical body. As your psychic abilities develop, all benefits will come more easily. They are an important part of your foundation for Psychic Anatomy Yoga.

Yoga has become and is still growing in popularity in North America. Its asanas (postures and movements) help strengthen and lengthen the body, so physical fluids and PE can move threw it more easily. Psychic Anatomy Yoga takes asanas a few steps further, including exercises for your psychic anatomy and

---

[10] I commented on the importance of self-help techniques in the preface.

14

some key psychic energy techniques with them. This enhances the benefits of yoga asanas[11] and in return, the asanas enhance the benefits of these exercises and techniques.

The reasons for these enhanced benefits involve how your psychic anatomy and physical body are interconnected (this is the mind-body-spirit connection). You may have heard something about your psychic anatomy before. It includes your aura[12] and its auric bodies and chakras, your meridians and vessels[13] (also known as nadis), your hara and its tan tiens, and your core star; all discussed in Chapters 3-7.

These parts of you are invisible to your five senses, but visible to your sixth sense, which is also known as Extra Sensory Perception[14] (ESP) or Clairvoyance. I'll give you a few examples of situations when you might have been aware of PE with your ESP. Do you recall feeling someone staring at you? Knowing who was calling or at your door before answering? Getting a sensation from a person, place or thing and having a knowing of what that sensation meant? These are all examples of your psychic anatomy, specifically your sixth and seventh chakras (discussed in Chapter 4) sensing PE.

Your psychic anatomy is very closely connected to your emotions, mind and spirit. This is why you feel with your ESP and sometimes have mental awareness as well. Psychic Anatomy Yoga helps strengthen your psychic anatomy, making you more emotionally and mentally aware of PE, which also helps you sense the probably future as these energies are not bound by time the same way physical matter is[15].

These are very big benefits to the decision rich lifestyles many people lead. In financial situations, life choices and sports,

---

[11] In the cases involving PE, this enhancement is very significant.
[12] Scientifically observable. See my book *The Psychic Energy Reality* for details.
[13] Scientifically observable. See my book *The Psychic Energy Reality* for details.
[14] Scientifically studied. See my book *The Psychic Energy Reality* for details.
[15] See Section 1 of *The Psychic Energy Reality* for several studies confirming this.

getting a sense of the probable future and being able to read between the lines of what people say/write/do or do not say/write/do can help us greatly.

This emotional and mental awareness plays into your intuition as well. Your intuition comes from your soul/higher-self and/or spirit guides as PE that you emotionally and/or mentally become aware of. Intuition can deliver superior guidance to anything you can comprehend as a human (in general). I mentioned previously that PE are not bound by time the same way physical material is, your soul and spirit guides have the same freedom and other advantages that they share with you as intuition.

Strengthening your psychic anatomy also comes with the benefits of being able to control PE for healing and empowering purposes more easily. This can be used in many ways to help yourself, as well as others live to your/their fullest potential.

Depending on your mind-body-spirit makeup, certain benefits will come faster than others. Common ones are long lasting relaxation, mental and emotional clarity, improved memory, self-awareness, ESP and blissful states of consciousness that get more powerful and longer lasting the more you practice.

Healing from chronic conditions is a powerful benefit that usually takes time. Chronic conditions are usually the result of large pockets of unhealthy PE that have gotten so strong over time that they oppress the physical body and can even change DNA[16]. With Psychic Anatomy Yoga, these pockets can be treated more directly than trying to treat the physical symptoms associated with them. Treating symptoms just slows it down. Treating the cause heals the condition.

---

[16] A possible example is hereditary diseases; the science is still developing. See *The Interface Between Psychic Energies and the Physical Body* and *The Psychic Energy Reality* for discussions.

16

Remember, PE are controlled and empowered by your attention, whether it is given internally (ex. your own thoughts and emotions) or external (ex. things happening around you). Focus your attention on the positive things you want more in your life, while still acknowledging and dealing with the negative ones[17]. This will make it easier to enjoy your life and life to your fullest potential. Enjoy the journey :) .

---

[17] *Inner and Outer Success* discusses the best of convention self-help techniques and several psychic energy techniques.

CHAPTER 2
THE VERY BEGINNING

The very beginning of all psychic energy practices is the meditative state. The meditative state is a calm, relaxed and comfortable state of mind, emotion and body. In this state, your brain's base vibration slows down and your body responds similarly. As your meditative state deepens, your brain continues to slow down, towards a base vibration where dreams occur (7.8 Hz[18]). Most people have their intense meditative experiences, visions and insights near 7.8 Hz.

PE and intuition are easier to use when you are in a meditative state, because your mind and emotions (psychic anatomy) are calmer, which are your tools for working with PE and intuition.

Reaching a meditative state just takes the intention to do so, but sometimes a little help goes a long way. Posture, breathing exercises, visualizations, affirmations, music, aromas (aromatherapy[19]) and sacred space are all effective techniques for helping you achieve and deepen your meditative state; discussed below.

In regular yoga practices, the meditative state is to be maintained during your entire practice. The same is true in Psychic Anatomy Yoga, and is even more important to do so, because it helps you become aware and work with PE and your intuition.

---

[18] Hz = cycles/second or beats/second.
[19] Discussed again in Level 8.

Posture

Sitting or standing in a comfortable, posture-correct position makes it easier for your psychic anatomy and physical body to function. Below is a description of posture-correct sitting and standing postures. If you had bad posture for awhile, it may take some time before you are comfortable in these postures. If this is the case, you would likely benefit from visiting a posture therapist and/or having a regular yoga asana practice.

There could also be psychic energy memories oppressing your posture. Slouched shoulders and a hanging head are examples of psychic energy memories associated with depression. Riskind et al, 1982, discusses a study of deliberate postures biasing people towards related emotions. Example, slouch and depressed postures in general bias participants towards helplessness in helplessness tests compared to those placed in expansive, upright postures. Every part of us is interconnected[20]!

Sitting Posture

Have your legs straight in front of you, uncrossed and with a 90-degree bend at the knees. Square your hips, comfortably straighten your spine (very important) and lift your chest slightly. Relax your shoulders back and down so they rest directly above your hips, jaw parallel with the ground and relaxed. Place your hands on your lap, palms facing up, down, towards each other[21] or resting with one hand in the other palm. You can also have them resting by your side, palms facing forward or inward. All positions have their advantages as discussed below.

---

[20] More on this subject within *The Psychic Energy Reality*.
[21] Common in many of the Psychic Anatomy Exercises.

With your palms facing up, you are in a better position for receiving PE and letting them wash down around and threw you, which is a form of cleansing. If you choose, you can lift your hands so you have a 90-degree bend at your elbows or above your head to increase the power of this cleansing posture (figures 2 and 3). Having a 90-degree bend has the advantage of being close to your fourth/heart chakra, which helps you connect to the PE you are working with; fourth/heart chakra discussed in Chapter 4. It is very common to naturally find your way into this positions when meditating and praying. Often these postures are associated with swaying or rocking back and forth as the PE increase in power.

When your palms are facing forward you are in a better posture for letting PE wash around and threw you (figure 4 and 5 (shows with standing)). The reason for this is that sending them directly into the Earth can slow them down. Faster flows can carry more away. Remember to have the intent of the released unhealthy PE being recycled by the Earth and/or vegetation so they are not left lingering in your environment. House plants are great for eating up unhealthy PE by the way.

When resting one hand in the palm of the other, you create a circuit that allows PE to circulate more easily within you. This helps empower the healthy PE you have/are receiving (figure 6). PE can be greatly intensified in the space between your hands, which is an important concept for the psychic energy exercises in general. When your palms face each other, PE can circulate within your body as well as your psychic anatomy more easily. If you choose, you can position your hands and arms so they make a circle involving your chest. This will empower the circulating energies even more. These last two options become more common in upper levels as a General Technique called Holding; General Techniques discussed below.

When hands are on your lap, palms facing down, you are more connected to your physical body, which is good for connecting and empowering yourself with Earth energies (figure 7). Resting your hands by your side is similar, except your hands can now help connect you to the Earth (figure 8).

Kneeling Stools

Kneeling is an excellent way to maintain a straight spine while sitting. Unfortunately, it can restrict circulation threw your legs, which is unhealthy. Sitting with crossed legs is another option, but it makes it hard to maintain a straight spine. Often it results in slouching, which is unhealthy as well.

Kneeling stools, also known as Meditation or Prayer Stools, can help in both postures. They take the weight off your legs when kneeling, allowing blood to flow threw them more easily (see figure 6). They also help raise your hips above your knees when sitting with crossed legs, which makes it easier to keep a straight spine (see figure 5). I find this the most comfortable way to sit on a kneeling stool.

When kneeling or sitting with crossed legs, you can use a foam or wooden yoga block as well. This is sometimes enough, although not always as comfortable as a kneeling stool, especially when kneeling!

In Appendix H, I present a simple and sturdy kneeling stool design that you can make yourself. Eventually, kneeling stools might be sold from the website as well.

Standing Posture

Have your feet shoulder width a part, hips squared and directly above your feet. Lift your chest slightly and relax your shoulders back and down to be above your hips. Comfortably straighten your spine (very important), jaw parallel with the ground and relaxed. You can rest your arms at your sides, palms facing forward, facing each other, facing up with the options discussed in siting posture or facing your body, wherever you feel drawn to place them. Sometimes you will feel the need to hold your hands in several different positions or to perform some movements with them. Trust your intuition when you have these insights, because this is how the masters practice.

When meditation requires you to stay in these postures for long periods of time, pressure can build up in your joints and muscles, especially if your body is not used to being in these postures. Allow yourself to move in smooth waving motions to help bring comfort to your body without disturbing your meditative state. I give more examples of such movements in Level 4 within *Psychic Anatomy* Exercises as Smooth Movements[22]. For purpose of this book, the asanas should help keep you comfortable on their own. Feel free to explore and be intuitive with Smooth Movements if you choose. They can be compared to intuitive dance.

You always have the option of changing your posture while in a meditative state, such as from standing to kneeling or sitting. As long as you move slowly and keep you spine erect, you should be able to easily maintain your meditation as you move.

---

[22] Smooth Movements are very common in qi-gong practices.

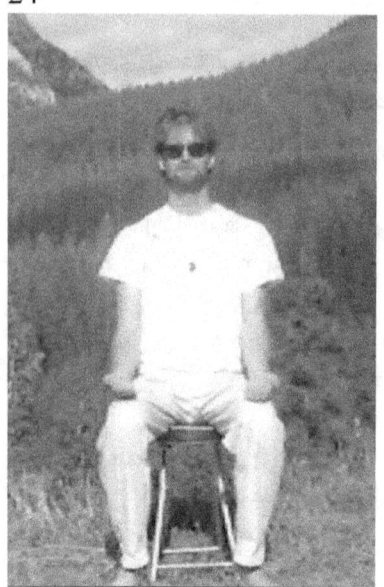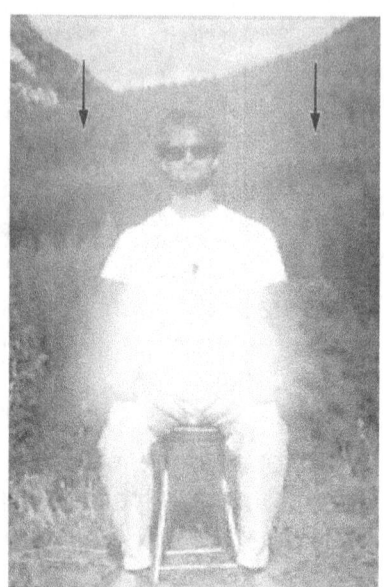

Figure 1: You can see the PE coming down from above and how they are more intense at the hands in the figure on the right.

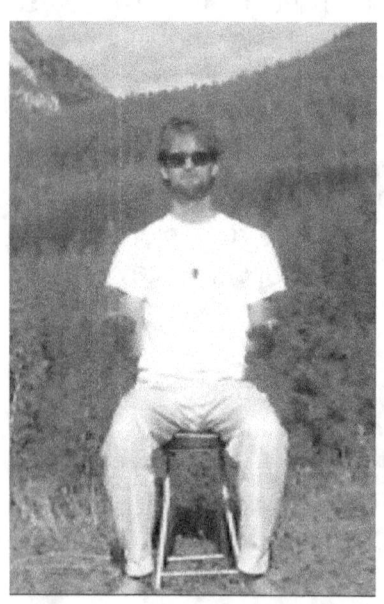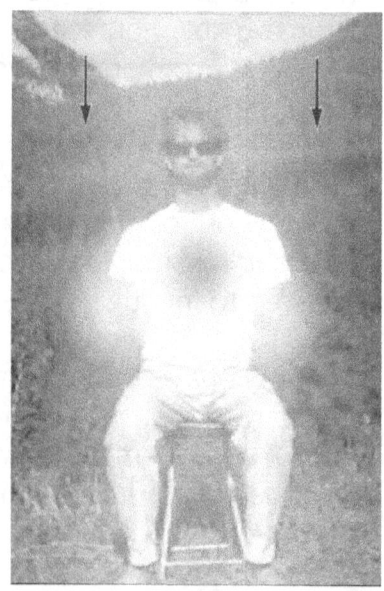

Figure 2: The green glow is the fourth/heart chakra responding to the increased intensity of PE. Chakras discussed in Chapter 4 and periodically in this book.

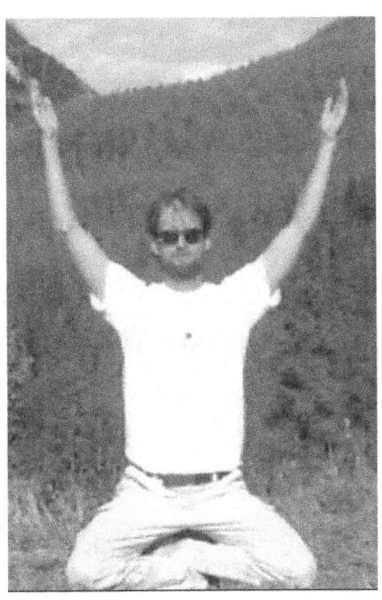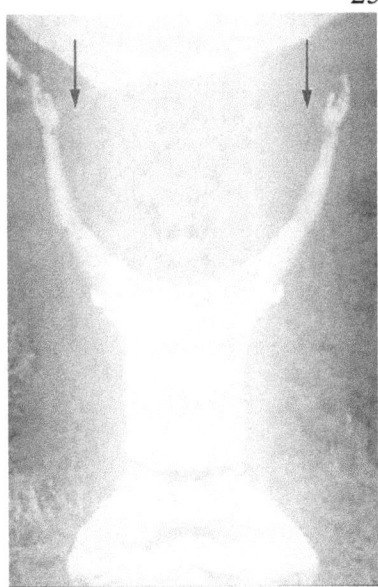

Figure 3: Shows a Kneeling Stool sitting posture, which is very good for keeping your spine straight for long periods on time.

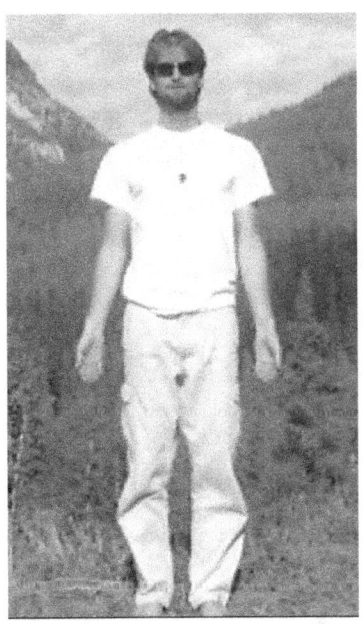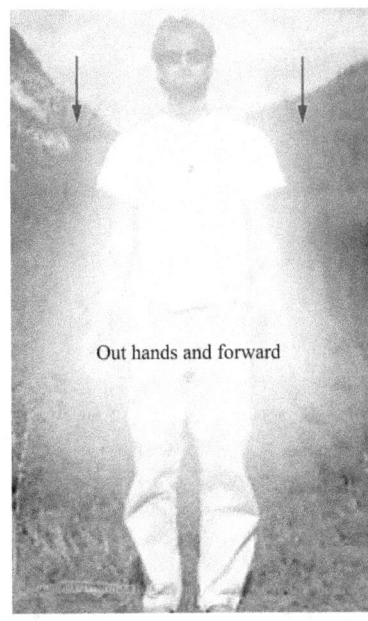

Out hands and forward

Figure 4: The figure on the right shows how palms direct flow of PE forward.

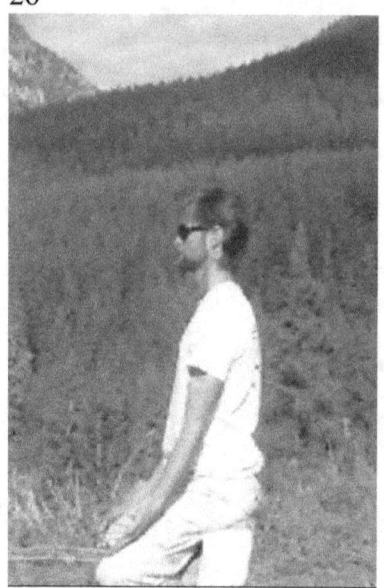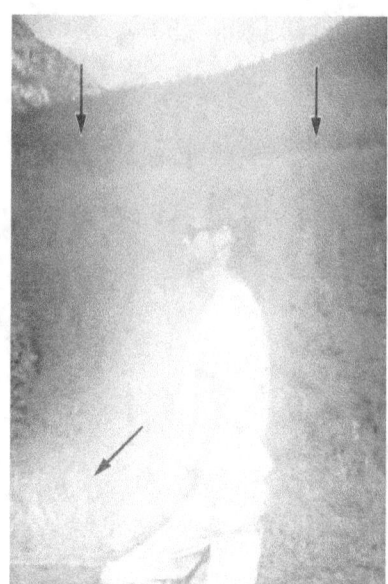

Figure 5. Shows a different posture on a Kneeling Stool and how the palms help bias the flow forward.

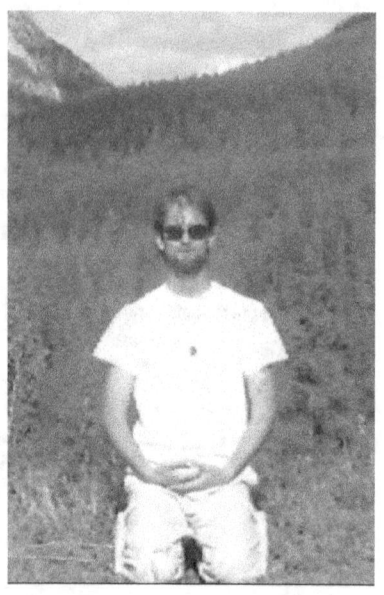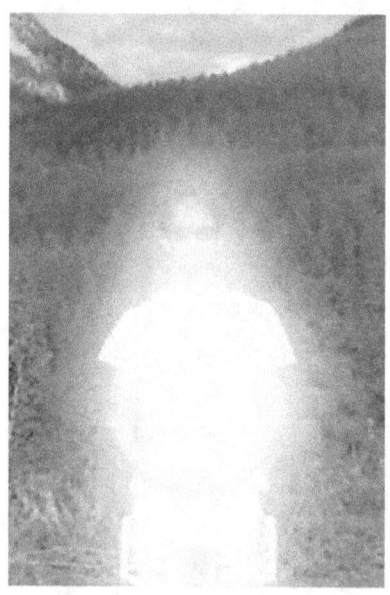

Figure 6: Shows the front view of the Kneeling Stool posture of figure 5. This hand position is very comfortable to incubating in healthy PE :) :) .

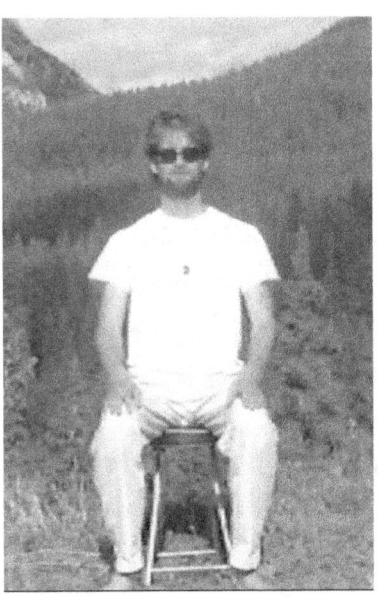 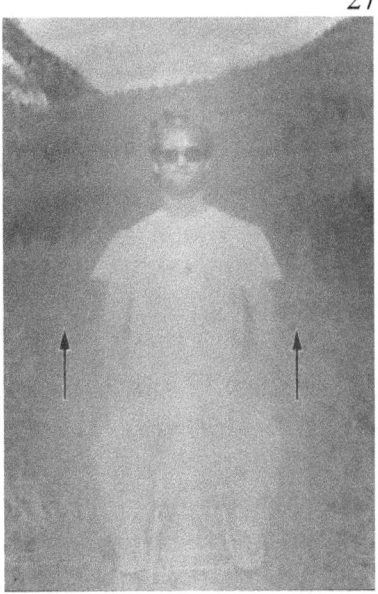

Figure 7: Placing your hands on your lap empowers the lower parts of your psychic anatomy. You can see the Earth PE (discussed below) are brighter there.

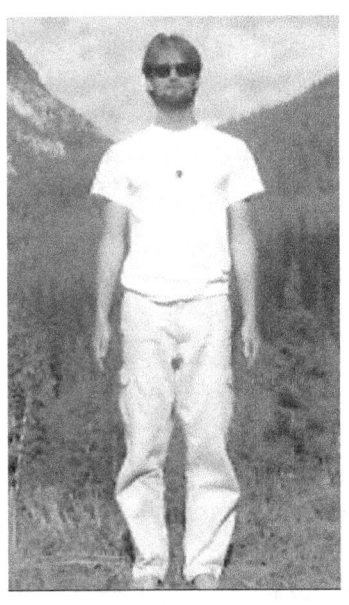 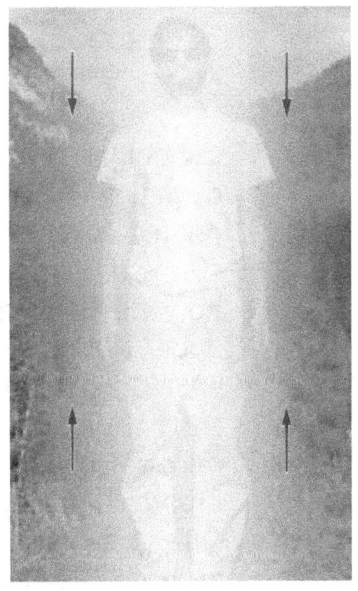

Figure 8: Makes your psychic anatomy narrower and more aligned for Conducting Heaven and/or Earth (discussed below).

Breath

Breath is emphasized as a very important technique for achieving and deepening meditative states in almost all meditative practices. Caponigro, 2005 reviews the teachings of breath in these practices, complimenting them with his own observations and techniques from his breath-healing practice and retreats.

In general, rhythmic breathing, which has equal times and tensions for inhalation and exhalation, and split second transitions between them, is considered healthy breathing. Progressively allowing your breathing to slow down and deepen in this way will help you go deeper into a meditative state. This will be called Circular or Healthy Breathing for the rest of this book.

Comments on Caponigro's book, *The Miracle of Breath*

Caponigro shares his perspectives on how deviations from healthy breathing are related to emotional/mental responses and states of being. For example, he describes how he has helped many people manage anger, anxiety, fear, stress and shock, as well as heal from disorders arising from suppression of these emotions of major and minor accounts by teaching them how to breath healthily while experiencing them. Often he will facilitate the release of associated unhealthy PE from muscles and the somatic nervous system as this happens.

When suppressed emotional PE get sufficiently strong, they can result in respiratory disorders, chronic pain, neuromuscular problems, psychotic breaks, schizophrenia, obsessive compulsive disorder, chronic anxiety and more. Catching patterns in your or someone else's breathing in response to unhealthy experiences can help a lot. When this happens, just focus (or help them focus) on healthy breathing to reduce the amount of unhealthy PE you/they take on and produce.

The main reason why controlled breathing, and meditation in general, have so many benefits is that the bioelectromagnetic signals of breathing in these ways is more balanced, harmonized and coherent. The heart and brain synchronize with the breathing patterns, which makes them more balanced, harmonized and coherent as well. This combination plays an important role in coordinating the bioelectromagnetic processes in the whole body, which as you can imagine becomes more balanced, harmonized and coherent, increasing general health and performance[23]. The more you maintain healthy breathing patterns, the more you reinforce these benefits.

---

[23] More on bioelectromagnetism in *The Interface Between Psychic Energies and The Physical Body, Becoming Super Human* and to a lesser degree in *The Psychic Energy Reality* and the research group called HeartMath.

Chest and Abdominal Breathing

Chest breathing is the most common form of breathing, which is healthiest when the entire rib cage expands and contracts equally in all directions. Focus on having your chest expand back, up, down and front as you breathe. It can release tension that has formed from lack of use if you have chronically not expanded your ribs in specific directions. Try this now. It will oxygenate your blood making it easier to read.

Abdominal and chest/abdominal breathing helps pump blood threw your body and move food threw your digestive system. For an internet based list of better breathing benefits, see the link in this footnote[24].

Visualization and Affirmations

Remember reading that everything you give your attention to, whether it is an emotion, thought or external experience, attracts associated PE to you? As you focus on becoming calm, relaxed and comfortable, you are attracting those PE to you and they influence you to become more calm, relaxed and comfortable. Your intention to feel calm, relaxed and comfortable is the main part, but focusing on thoughts and emotions associated with being so, using things like memories, visualizations and/or affirmations can empower your intentions greatly. These are different ways of focusing attention.

You may find that one or a combinations of these techniques work best for you. I find memories to be the most powerful, because they are more direct. They reference psychic energy memories associated with the PE attempting to be attracted, and doing so helps strengthen them as well, making them more powerful aspects of your subconsciousness.

---

[24]   www.breathing.com/articles/benefits.htm

As you evolve, your potential will exceed your memories, but still focusing on them can serve as foundation for your potential to exceed them, creating new memories to reference in the future.

Making use of multiple techniques is ultimately the most effective, because it is more comprehensive. Remember that as you use the same techniques to achieve relaxation and other states of consciousness, their associated psychic energy memories grow, making it easier to stay and return to these states. This is an example of the power of rituals. Remember that rituals need to be broken as better ones are discovered.

Heartmath is a research group that has a lot of success using visualizations and affirmations while focusing on the heart to empower meditative states and peoples abilities to use PE, specifically for energy healing purposes [Heartmath, INT1]. Your heart is the strongest electromagnetic signal in your body, which makes it important for tuning into PE physically[25].

Here are some example affirmations I call the Fundamental Affirmations.

---

[25] This is discussed again in Level 5.

Fundamental Affirmations

1) I only allow PE within and around me that are for my personal and our collective evolution.

2) I call back all PE that I have focused away from myself that are not being used for my personal and our.

3) I release all unhealthy PE from within and around me with the intent that they be recycled by the Earth and/or vegetation. You can visualize a waterfall or channel of white light washing these PE away.

4) I accept all healthy PE that empower me in the direction of my personal and our collective evolution.

Music

Music has always been a popular way to relax, unwind and meditate. I've found many New Age CDs that are great for meditation, but I also like CDs with more dramatic sounds of spiritual/emotional context, which create power during a meditation as PE move around and release in harmony with the music.

There are also Brain Entrainment or Brain Synchronization CDs available that use audio frequencies to facilitate your brain's base vibration to enter the meditative state. The Monroe

Institute and Holosync are leaders in using Bilateral Beats to reach these deep states of meditation, while balancing left and right brain hemispheres[26]. There is also software on the internet for making your own; some of it being free.

Similar things can be done with electromagnetic waves that have a lot of additional health benefits. I discuss this in more depth within *Becoming Super Human.* You can also learn more online with the key word Pulsed Electromagnetic Frequencies (PEMF).

Sacred Space

Practicing Psychic Anatomy Yoga, Psychic Anatomy Exercises/Treatments or any practice involving PE, is best done in a sacred space. Sacred spaces make it easier to attract healthy PE and maintain their presence. Any space came be made into a sacred space, all you need to do is treat them like an alter. Bless your sacred space(s), focusing your attention on empowering, balancing and harmonizing them with healthy PE and clearing away unhealthy PE. Affirmations, visualizations, gemstones and aromatherapy and more can all help.

Meditation

Meditative practices have increased in popularity since I first began working with PE in 1995. Mindfulness, Emptiness and other Asian concepts attract a verity of people in North America. Although there are many different names for meditation, there are essentially only two forms. Emptiness, which is when you empty your awareness by ignoring everything that enters it. The other is Focused Meditation, which is when you focus your

---

[26] The left and right side of your brain needs to work together for many functions. See Munroe, INT1, for more information.

attention on something specific, such as an affirmation, visualization or attracting healthy PE.

Experiential/Vision Meditations are a combination of emptiness and focused meditation. In them, you focus your attention on becoming aware of what you are experiencing/visions. The role of emptiness is to allow information to drift threw[27] your awareness until you choose to focus upon something, such as PE, parts of your psychic anatomy or a vision.

Experiential Meditation

Experiential Meditation can be done at any time during a Psychic Anatomy Yoga practice, as well as on its own, such as before going to bed. It is used in Psychic Anatomy Yoga for reflecting on your experiences, observing thoughts, emotions, PE, allowing visions to unfold and most importantly, to integrate and harmonize with the PE you have attracted and worked with during your practice. Integrating and harmonizing simply takes the intent to do so while in a meditative state, although there are some specific techniques that I will discuss.

I recommend spending some time getting familiar with what has been discussed so far. It will help you create a good foundation for the rest of this chapter and book. You may also be able to intuitively build upon this information, being content with your practice for several weeks and maybe even months. As I have already stated and I will state periodically in the rest of this book, intuition is your greatest tool. Trust it, develop it.

General Techniques

There are nine general techniques that will be discussed below.

---

[27] I use the word "threw" intentionally.

They appear in several figures and are shown periodically in the DVDs[28]. The first five all use your hands. Your hands have very strong psychic anatomy, which makes them powerful tools for working with PE. Their strength comes from how much you use them to express yourself, which causes PE to flow threw and around them.

The simplest General technique is holding your hands over the area you are working with to intensify the PE there; this is called Holding (figure 9). Another is a powerful modification of Holding, called Pulsating (figure 10 and 11). Pulsating has your hands expanding away from and coming back to the area you are working with repeatedly. You can visualize healthy PE flushing in and out of the area, helping to loosen and remove unhealthy PE as healthy PE take their place. When these movements are timed with your breathing, it is called Pulsate Breathing.

There are two ways to do Pulsate Breathing. You can either expand your hands away as you inhale, visualizing the area you are working with expanding as it breathes in healthy PE. When exhaling, bring your hands back towards this area, visualizing it contracting as it releases unhealthy PE. The other approach is to pull out unhealthy PE as you expand on the exhale and pushing in healthy PE as you inhale. The slower you do these techniques the more effective they will be.

The fourth technique is called Spinning. Spinning is used in several psychic energy practices to help amplify PE. Having the intention to Spin PE causes them to Spin. Moving your hands in a circular motion helps them Spin. In general, clockwise Spins encourage PE to away from you, while counter-clockwise Spins move towards you. This can be used to help empower the flow of PE in the Heaven and Earth Exercises; these exercise are discussed below.

---

[28] Discussed in the Other Books & DVDs by Brett A. Rogers near the end of this book.

The fifth technique is called Expanding. Pulsate techniques can be used to help expand your psychic anatomy by not contracting all the way back to your original state, resulting in more and more expansion as you Pulsate Breathe. You can also just use your intent, which gets easier as you get more powerful at working with PE and your psychic anatomy. In an expanded state, PE can move more easily, making it easier for unhealthy ones to be released and healthy ones to be brought in. PE can also expand, which makes them more sensitive to resonance with PE of a higher vibration (ex. PE associated with higher consciousness). Expanding can be done on a very small scale, such as the aura of your DNA ,to a very large scale such as your entire being. Usually it will be your entire being that is Expanding.

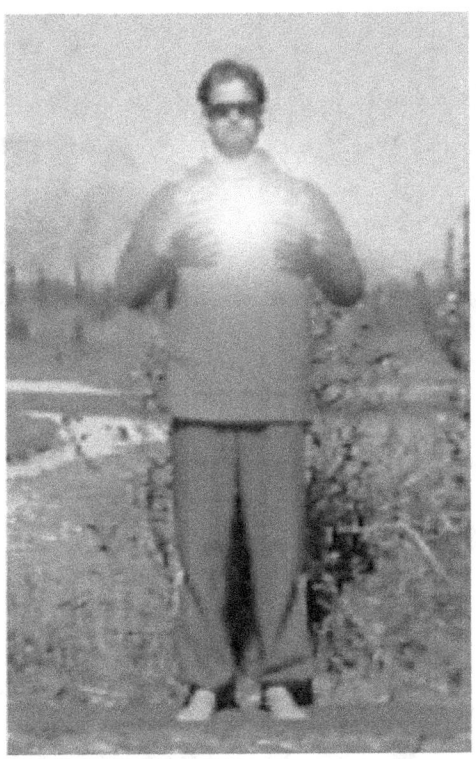

Figure 9. Shows Holding a ball of PE. This is an important concept for concentrating PE; expanded upon In Chapters 4-7. Pulsate techniques are important concepts for a similar reason.

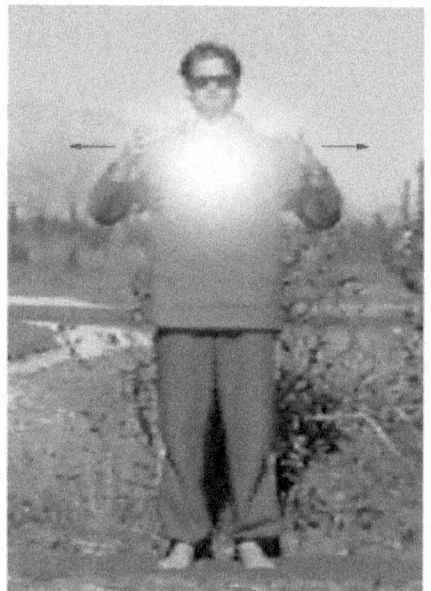 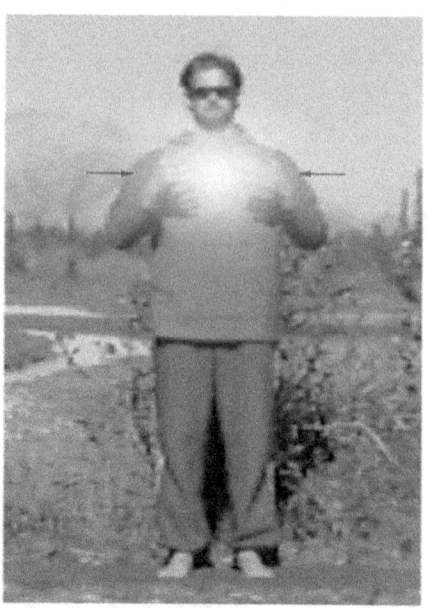

Figure 10: Expand on the inhale (left) and contract on the exhale (right).

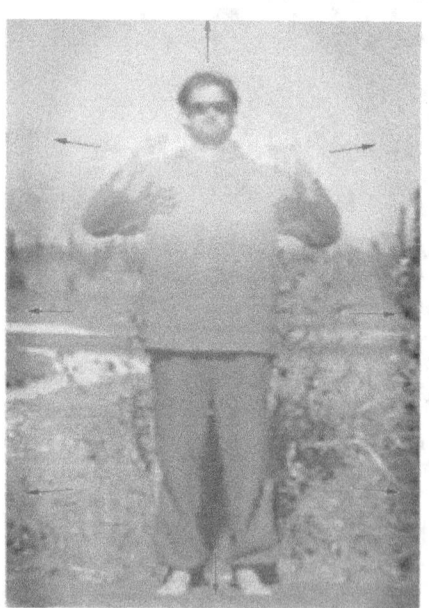 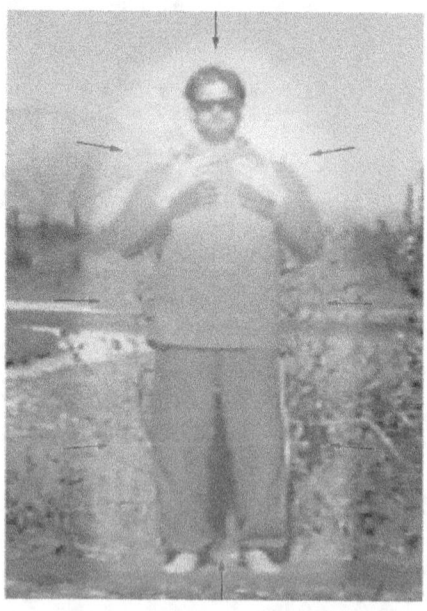

Figure 11: On the left you can see my knees are straight and on the right they are slightly bent. My spine does something similar to physically contract and expand. Psychic anatomy and the physical body are interconnected.

The sixth technique comes in handy when PE are being released. It is called Sweeping (figure 12-14). The idea is to sweep your hands over the area you are working with to sweep away the PE being released. Usually this techniques is combined with the intention for the released PE to be recycled by the Earth and/or vegetation.

Scanning is the seventh technique (figure 15 and 16), which is very similar to Sweeping, but the movements are slower, and your intention is to scan the areas you are moving over and/or help circulate PE. Scanning is commonly done by moving your hands up and down in front of your body with both hands together or separately. This is a very common technique in traditional qi-gong practices. It is a great technique to help get you tuned into yourself to start your practice and during.

Sometimes you will be intuitively guided to do specific things that are out of sequence with your/the group's[29] routine. These intuitive insights are very important and can guide you to do almost anything. Trusting them is the eigth technique called Intuitive Movements. As you advance in your practice, it will become more commonly used.

Grounding is the ninth technique that is highly recommended to do periodically during and especially after your practice. It will help integrate and strengthen the new state of your psychic anatomy, making you feel more centered, balanced and in control. Visualizing roots coming from your feet and going into the Earth as you connect to the Earth Is a very popular and effective technique.

When connected to the Earth, you can draw upon Earth energies to help ground and empower yourself; this is discussed in more detail in Chapter 10 with respect to the Heaven and Earth Exercises. Another great way to get grounded is to do

---

[29] Practicing with a group has a lot of advantages; discusses in Appendix A.

physical things, such as working with plants, walking in nature, exercising and more. Do what works for you.

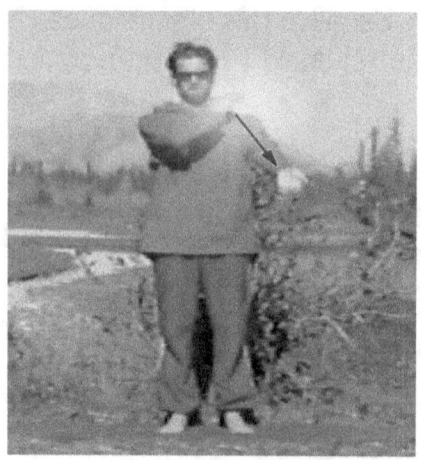 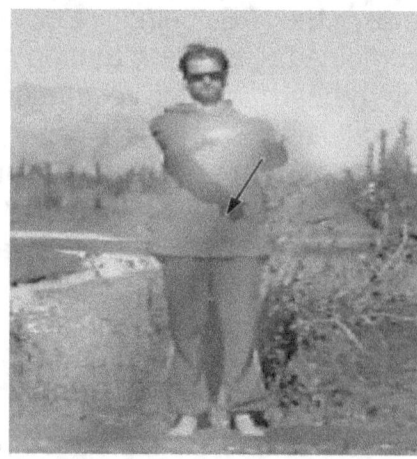

Figure 12: Remember to Sweep with the intent of the unhealthy PE being recycled by the Earth and/or vegetation. The darkness within the light is intended to be unhealthy PE being released.

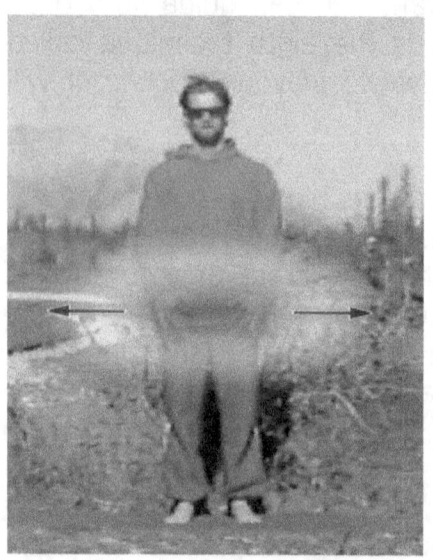 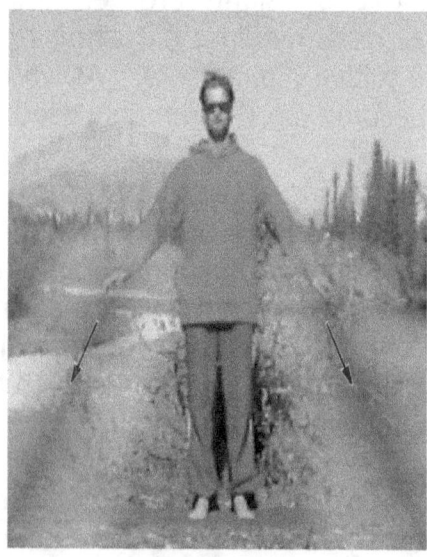

Figure 13: A simple example of how Holding and/or Pulsating techniques can resulting in unhealthy PE surfacing for release that release easily. In the next set of figures, two situations are shown of unhealthy PE that are harder to release (parts a-e) and when there is a lot being released (part f).

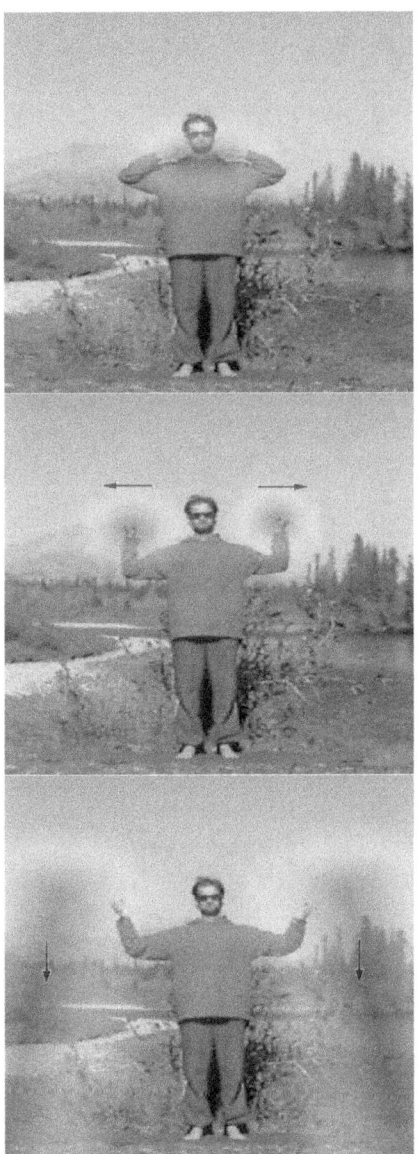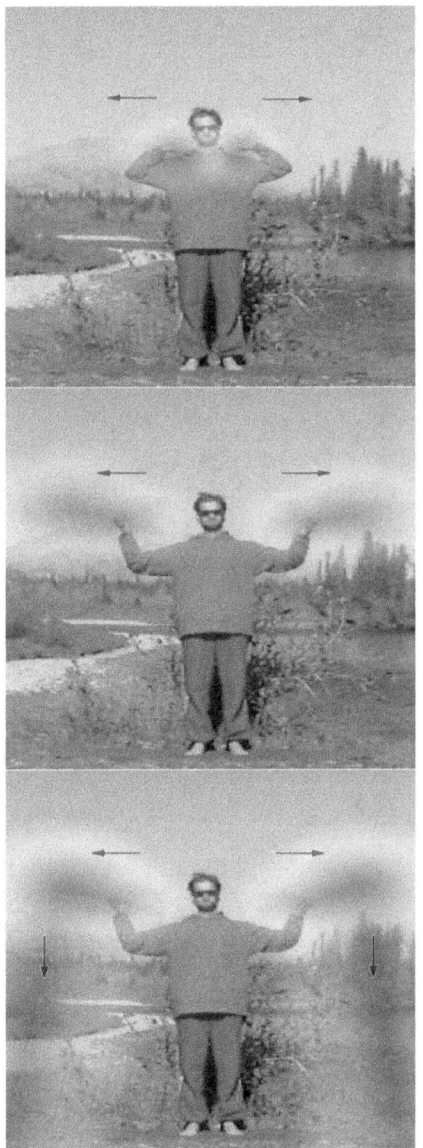

Figure 14: Flows from the top left (part a) to the top right (part b) and so on. Part a shows unhealthy PE being gathered. How long it takes for this gathering to occur is a sense you will develop. Usually its quiet short. Part b shows them being pulled away. Part c shows how they are grabbed onto and then released in part d. Part e shows how the intent of sending them into the Earth for recycling manifests. Part f is when a lot of unhealthy PE keep coming out. When this happens, be patient and let them flow.

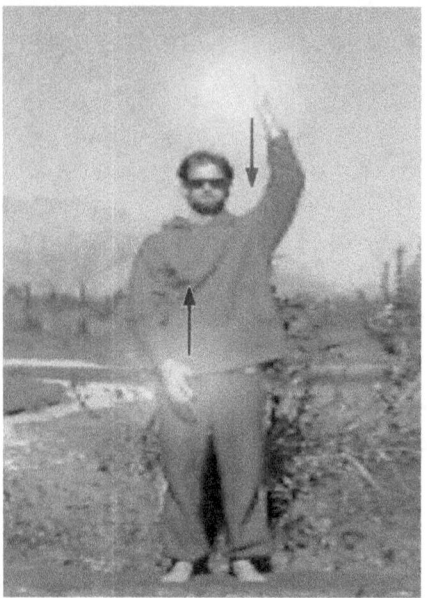 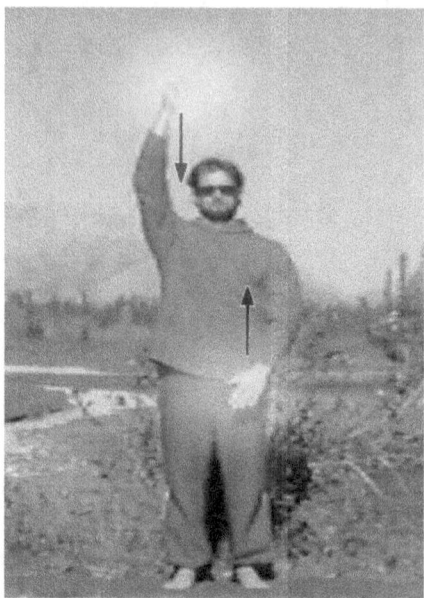

Figure 15: Scanning with hands moving in opposite directions, which can be timed with your breath.

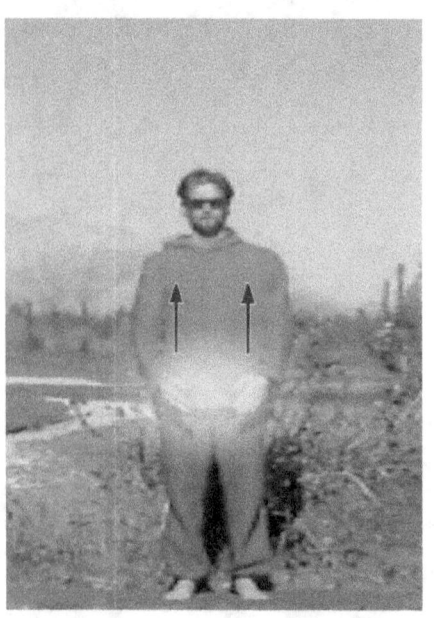 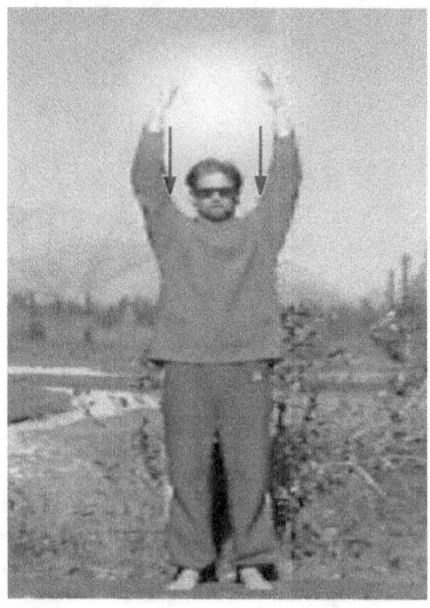

Figure 16: Scanning with hands moving together, which can also be timed with your breath.

General Techniques
Holding
Pulsating
Pulsate Breathing
Spinning
Expanding
Sweeping
Scanning
Intuitive Movements
Grounding

Warm-up Routine

Before doing the psychic energies exercises in this book, it is a good idea to do some stretching and general relaxation to help loosen our physical body and get into a meditative state. This makes it easier for PE to flow within you. Yoga asanas are a great warm-up routine.

Preparation Exercises

Note: Before getting into these preparation exercises, remember that they will be described as simple as possible first and then be expanded upon immediately following the simple description. Just take them to the depth of complexity you are comfortable with and return to them when you are ready to go more into depth.

Preparation exercises are the first thing done before at all psychic energy practices. They help clear your psychic anatomy and environment of loosely held unhealthy PE, empower the healthy ones and increase balance and harmony. They can be done in a number of ways for any amount of time. Even a few seconds can make a noticeable difference, especially as you develop. The best preparation exercises for beginners are

Pulsate Breathing and Scanning; discussed below.

The Fundamental Affirmations are great preparation exercises for beginners and experienced people as well. Focus on each affirmation and give yourself time for the PE associated with them to do their thing before moving onto the next. Remember that affirmations are for focusing your attention, simply saying them is not enough.

Rewording them for your environment can also be done after doing them on yourself. An example of this rewording is below.

Fundamental Affirmations for an Environment

1) I only allow PE within and around this environment (ex. sacred space, home or place of work) that contribute to my personal and our collective evolution.

2) I release all unhealthy PE from within and around this environment with the intent that they be recycled by the Earth and/or vegetation. You can visualize a waterfall or channel of white light washing these energies away.

3) I accept and empower all healthy PE into and around this environment that contribute to my personal and our collective evolution.

Preparation exercises are to make the healthy PE and psychic energy memories in your psychic anatomy and environment more dominant, balanced and harmonized making it easier for you to attract healthy PE. Beginners should take at least fifteen minutes to practice these affirmation exercises effectively. It will give you a good chance to experience them. Once you start to notice them working, it will be well worth the effort, also it will make it easier to use them in the future. Doing them with a group can greatly help empower them as well; see Appendix A for more on group practice.

Here are three examples of how important preparation is. In Schwartz, 2007, p. 140, E-Coli bacteria injured by heat stress were given Reiki treatments. It was found that stressed practitioners further induced injury, while healthier practitioners helped them recover[30]. This study was extended to include a 15-minute pretreatment to a person[31], which helped the practitioners get into a healthier state. This significantly improved E-Coli recovery responses.

Braith, 1988, and Shapiro, 1992, are studies on the adverse effects of meditation during significant influences of unhealthy PE (ex. chronic anxiety and emotional release).

Pulsate Breathing Exercise

This Pulsate Breathing Exercise (shown in figure 10) is a great preparation exercise. Its expansive and easy to do. It starts by entering a meditative state (recall posture correct postures and Circular Breathing). Focus on being calm, relaxed and comfortable, making use of memories, visualization and/or affirmations if you choose. When you are ready turn your hands to face each other.

---

[30] A questionnaire was used to get an idea of the practitioner's state of mind, body and spirit health and performance.

[31] Essentially a preparation exercise.

Expand the distance between your hands as you inhale with the intent of healthy PE filling the space between them (visualizing the PE as a ball of light helps). As you exhale, let your hands come closer together, compressing the healthy PE between them. Continue to do this as the charge of healthy PE builds.

Intuition could guide you to focus this charge upon certain parts of yourself or direct it somewhere in the room or at a distance. It is common for intuition to take over after doing this exercise for a while. I recommend a bit of Scanning to follow when you are ready.

Lots of people feel tingling, heat, coldness and other sensations in their hands and body from this exercise. These sensations are the result of your psychic anatomy and physical body responding to the PE. As you develop, your psychic anatomy and physical body will adjust (activate), making them less sensitive to PE in these ways and more sensitive as your Extrasensory Perception (ESP).

Full Body Pulsate Breathing Exercise

This Full Body Pulsate Breathing Exercise (shown in figure 11) is a step up from the Pulsate Breathing Exercise. By holding your hands in front of you and/or positioning your hands and arms so they make a smooth curve involving your chest, the ball of light from the Pulsate Breathing Exercise can be made to surround your physical body, merging with your psychic anatomy.

You can include the intentions of the ball absorbing healthy PE as you inhale and releasing unhealthy PE as you exhale. You can also do it in reverse, for unhealthy PE to be pulled out as you inhale and healthy PE filling you as you exhale. I personally prefer the first way, but some people find the second way to be more natural. It is up to you, unless you are in a group. Group members contribute to the collective consciousness of the group and need to be coherent for optimal results. See Appendix A for more information on working with groups.

Both exercises can enhance your intuitive awareness, which is the a great benefit to these exercises, as well as life in general. Sometimes intuition will guide you to follow the exercises as they are taught precisely, especially in the beginning, but sometimes it will guide you to diverge. A common intuitive insight is to Sweep your hands over your body or threw your psychic anatomy to help PE release. Other common insights are to rub, shake, bounce and/or flick/kick a limb like you are sending a wave of PE threw and out of them. Throwing a wave can be considered a form of internal Sweeping for clearing out unhealthy PE. When you send a wave or Sweep out unhealthy PE, make sure you throw them into the Earth and/or vegetation with the intent of it being recycled. Directing unhealthy PE in this way can happen in group practice, which is an even more important time to be mindful of where you are sending them.

If you practice everything above for a few days, it will help build a good foundation for the rest of this book. Especially in the beginning, the Preparation Exercises should always be used as a warm-up for the exercises in the rest of this book.

48

CHAPTER 3
INTRODUCTION TO PSYCHIC ANATOMY

You already know that you are more than just a physical body. You have psychic anatomy that sends, receives and stores the PE associated with what you give your attention to. Whether it is your own thoughts and emotions, people, places or things, everything has PE associated with it.

In the following chapters, the four main parts of human psychic anatomy will be introduced briefly[32]. This information will teach about what your psychic anatomy does, how it works and what it looks like energetically. Having this knowledge will make it easier to become aware and work with it when practicing Psychic Anatomy Yoga.

Following the introduction to each psychic anatomy system, the essentials exercises involving them from the Psychic Anatomy Exercises will be taught[33], which you will learn to incorporate with yoga asanas in Section?.

Take your time with the information and exercises in this section. It will help develop a good foundation for proceeding exercises.

---

[32] *The Psychic Anatomy Exercises* goes into more depth and compliment this book. *The Psychic Energy Reality* goes into scientific detail about PE and psychic anatomy.

[33] The entire practice can be found within *The Psychic Anatomy Exercises.*

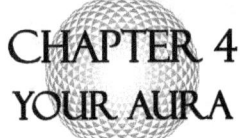

CHAPTER 4
YOUR AURA

The aura is probably the most popular part of human psychic anatomy. It can be found in many New Age books, spiritual teachings and scientific research[34]. Your aura consists of chakras and auric bodies. The chakras (shown in figure 17 as the circles and cones) are the parts that send and receive PE between you and other people, places and things. Each one works with certain types of PE; discussed below.

Your auric bodies (shown as concentric orbs in the figure 17) store the PE that you have given your attention to as psychic energy memories. These memories act as your unconscious mind, influencing you to focus your attention in ways that empower the psychic energy memories that are already apart of you. Hence, it is important to empower healthy PE and remove unhealthy ones. I will teach you ways to do this well[35].

Each auric body stores certain types of PE, which are the same as those for the chakras they are color coded with in figure 17. This is known as a region. Your first chakra and first auric body, color-coded red in the figures, works with the PE associated with physical survival. Your second chakra and second auric body work with the PE of emotions. The third with mental PE, the fourth with relationships and the fifth with expressions.

---

[34] Scientific research involving the aura has developed to the point where looking for evidence of its existence is no longer the main goal, we are now trying to better understand it. Discussed in *The Psychic Energy Reality.*

[35] For help with more powerfully imprinted psychic energy memories, see *Inner and Outer Success.*

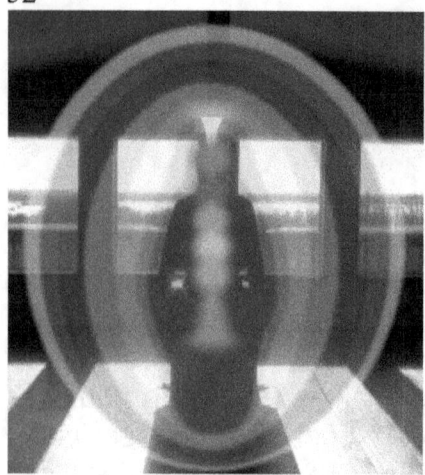 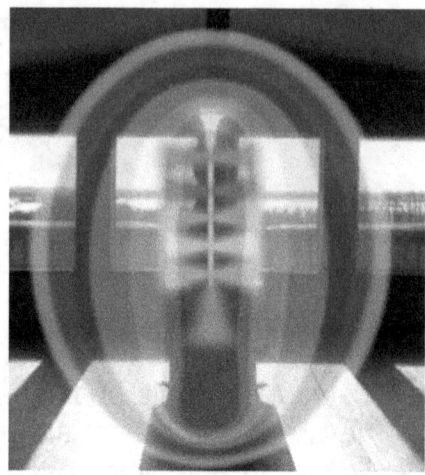

Figure 17: Shows the front view of the Human Aura on the left and a side view right.

Your sixth works with how PE feel (clairvoyance), similar to emotions, but the emotions are triggered by PE rather than your psychology. Your seventh works with mental awareness of PE (psychicism), which are thoughts triggered by PE. For example, if a person is having a thought and you become aware of the PE associated with that thought, you could have an emotional (feels happy) and/or mental response (they like what I said). Usually, such a response is the combination of the two, and a biasing of your psychology jumping to conclusions. The exercises in this book, as well as my other books, will help reduce this jumping to a conclusion part[36].

Table: Aura Facts

Chakra #	Chakra Name	Works with the PE of	# of Sub-chakras
1st	Root	Physical Survival and Life Force	4
2nd	Sacral	Emotions	8
3rd	Solar	Mind	10
4th	Heart	Relationship with Self and Others	12
5th	Throat	Expression	16
6th	Third eye	Emotional Awareness of PE	96
7th	Crown	Mental Awareness of PE	972

---

[36] *Inner and Outer Success* is the best book for this purpose.

The exercises that follow are the essential aura Psychic Anatomy Exercises[37]. In the beginning, it can take awhile for your awareness of what is happening during these exercises to develop. During this time, benefits can still be achieved. In the beginning of anyone's journey with practices involving PE, a lot can happen quickly, because they have never exercised this part of themselves before. This can result in change that used to take months, happening in a single session for some people!

Some people will have strong healing experiences, which can result in a fast release of unhealthy PE from their past. These experiences can sometimes be unsettling, but they are always extremely rewarding! An Energy Healing-Empowerment facilitator can induce and speed up such experiences, as well as enhance their quality. If you have a lingering unsettling experience, I recommend visiting an Energy Healing-Empowerment facilitator.

In the beginning, most people just feel warmth, tingling, mental clarity and pleasant feelings. As you develop, you can look forward to more profound experiences of increased mental and emotional health and performance. You can also look forward to being more clairvoyant, psychic and powerful at controlling PE.

The concept of these exercises is to focus your attention on the healthiest PE for each chakra one at a time. This can be done with just intention for it to happen as you focus your awareness on each chakra, but you can also include your hands, which empowers the exercises greatly.

---

[37] See *The Psychic Anatomy Exercises* for more.

Chakra Exercise 1

Turn your palms to face your first chakra in a standing or sitting posture. Focus your attention on the healthiest PE for this chakra as you focus upon it. If it feels appropriate, you can change from Holding to Pulsate, Pulsate Breathing, Sweep and/or Intuitive Movements. Remember that memories, affirmations and visualizations associated with the PE you want to empower will help empower them. For example, remembering[38] times when you felt really physically healthy or visualizing your chakra getting brighter and larger.

After the first chakra, move to your second chakra and then to you third and then fourth. I recommend five to twenty breaths (more is usually better) with each chakra before moving onto the next. When you are done with your fourth chakra, focus your attention on your chakras being balanced and harmonized individually and together.

Scanning can be used during this time as well. It can help you identify chakras that need extra attention. In the beginning this maybe hard for some people. If so, keep practicing and it will get easier.

Its OK to drift into an Experiential Meditation[39] for awhile after focusing on balancing and harmonizing your chakras. When you are ready, move onto Chakra Exercise 2.

---

[38] An even better, but more difficult approach for some people is focusing on the feeling of being healthy. This way you can focus on feeling healthier than you have ever felt.

[39] Recall that an Experiential Meditation is when you just witness/observe what you are feeling/thinking.

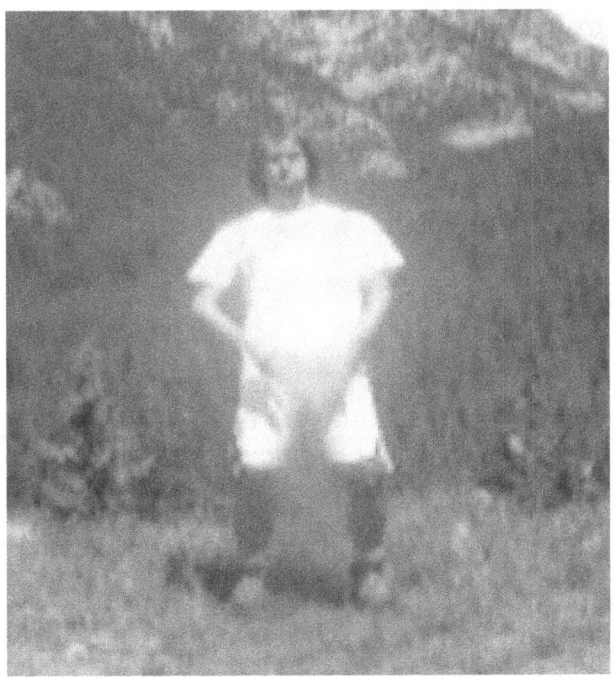

Figure 18: Shows the Scanning technique (double handed) being used at the end of Chakra Exercise 1.

Chakra Exercise 2

This is a progression from Chakra Exercise 1. From the fourth chakra or after balancing and harmonizing the fourth to first chakras, move to the fifth, sixth and then seventh, balancing and harmonizing the seventh to fourth at the end and then the seventh to first.

You can continue with this exercise as well, starting with your seventh chakra and working towards our first. Cycling up and down your chakras in this way is a good idea, because as improvements occur with one chakra, chakras you have already worked with could be affected, resulting in them being ready for more attention.

Cycling also involves the benefits of Ascending/Descending; discussed in Chapter 11.

It is best to keep practicing these exercises until you are comfortable with them, so you have a good foundation for the exercises to come.

Auric Body Exercise 1 and 2

This exercise follows the same pattern as the last two, except your attention is given to your auric bodies instead of chakras.

Sweeping, Scanning and Intuitive Movements are good techniques to use in your auric bodies. Intuitive Movements can include making sounds to resonant with PE and bouncing on the spot. Bouncing on the spot is a popular technique used in Asian practices, sometimes called "Cure for a Thousand Illnesses".

It is best to practice these exercises for a while before moving on to the meridian exercises in the next Chapter. As the health and performance of your aura improves, there will be more healthy PE for you to use in the meridian exercises.

Aura Exercise 1 and 2

Aura Exercise may be too advanced for some people at this point. If so, you can skip over it and return to it at a later date. It is a combination of the Chakra and Auric Body exercises.

You still use your hands to work with your chakras, but you include your auric bodies in your focused intent. For example, visualizing your fourth chakra and fourth auric body breathing with Pulsate Breathing. Visualizing it getting brighter and larger

(Expanding) as it fills with healthy PE.

I recommend incorporating the Full Body Pulsate Breathing Exercise as well. In this exercise, the bubble surrounding your body becomes an auric body (or several auric bodies as you progress).

When expanding and contracting auric fields with your breath, remember that you can place your arms to form a circle with your chest to empower these expansions and contractions (an application of geometry). As you breath in, allow the circle created with your arms to expand and as you exhale for it to contract. This will empower the expanding and contracting.

Scanning combines very well with this exercise. Even when breathing with one auric field and its color coded chakra, the interconnection between them and other parts of your psychic anatomy will make Scanning over them advantageous.

Yin-Yang

In general, Yin-Yang places one hand at the bottom of your reach, palm facing up towards your seventh chakra and your other hand at the top of your reach, palm facing towads your first chakra or up (figure 19). While in Yin-Yang, focus on there being balance and harmony within your chakra system and psychic anatomy in general.

Placing your hands at these two positions or on your seventh and first chakras directly for this purpose is commonly practiced in Energy Healing modalities and qi-gong. After spending at least 5 seconds (or minutes) with this intent, you can move one of your hands to just before your fourth chakra and focus on the four chakras between your hands being balanced and harmonized.

Reversing hands is usually done after repeating a series of asanas. For example, Warrior asanas with left leg forward then Warrior asanas with right leg forward. Note that when reversed, there will be three different chakras and your fourth chakra between your hands. Your fourth chakra is always included.

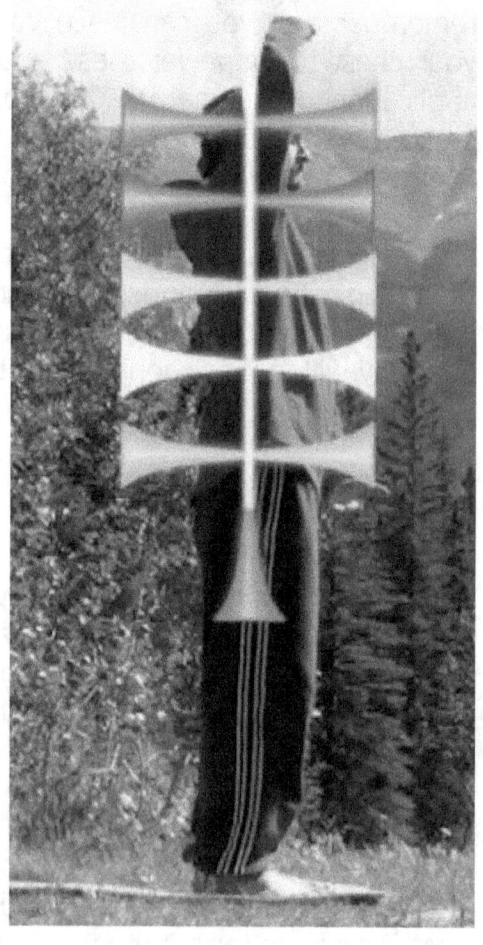

Figure 19: Shows Yin-Yang at the end of Chakra Exercise 2.

It is common for Yin-Yang to be used as a pause while Scanning. It can also be used for specific chakras (figure 20) or pairs of them. Yin-Yang can be used for any number of chakras, as well as any center of your psychic anatomy.

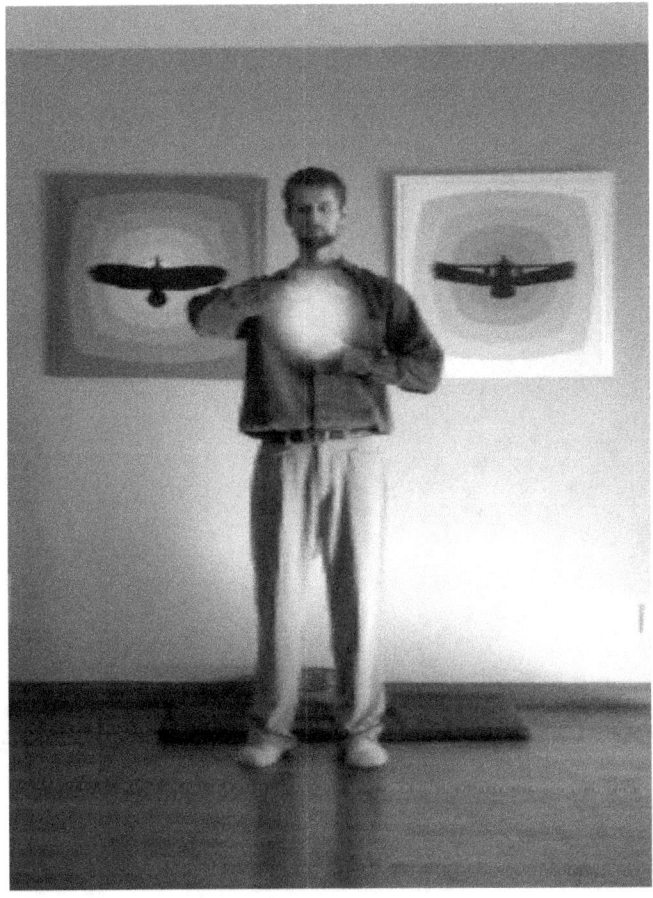

Figure 20: Shows Yin-Yang over just the fourth charka.

CHAPTER 5
YOUR MERIDIANS AND VESSELS

There are twelve meridians and eight vessels that help interface the PE in your aura and environment with your physical body[40]. Each meridian and vessel is believed to work with different types of PE and in different ways, but over the four thousand years of study, primarily coming from Traditional Chinese Medicine, there has never been an agreed upon conclusion to what these differences are.

There are some commonalities though. The meridians and vessels exist just under the skin[41] and all work with in a slightly different type of psychic energy, which is summarized in the descriptions below. By attracting and focusing healthy PE[42] threw your meridians and vessels with your mind and/or hands/finger tips[43], you can help expand and empower your meridians and vessels to free blockages and increase their general health and performance. Note that figures 21-34 have start and finish points for each meridian/vessel.

Another commonalty is that each meridian is paired with another. In the meridian descriptions below, paired meridians are placed in sequence (ex. Stomach Meridian and then the Spleen Meridian). I also comment on this pairing in the figure captions.

---

[40] This interface is discussed in scientific detail in my book *The Interface Between Psychic Energies and the Physical Body*.

[41] Lots of evidence supports this. See *The Psychic Energy Reality* and *The Interface Between Psychic Energies and the Physical Body* for details.

[42] The descriptions can help refine these healthy PE to be more specific to their function.

[43] A study I did on this technique is discussed on my website.

Working with your meridians is very rewarding, but it does take some discipline to memorize and become aware of them. Memorizing the path they take in your body is the first step. See figures 21-34. These vessels and meridians figures appear in the same order as their descriptions.

Yoga teachings often call meridians and vessels, Nadis. They only have a different name, because it comes from a different culture (Hinduism rather than Traditional Chinese Medicine). Some nadis have been identified as having very similar descriptions as the twelve major meridians as well as the Conception and Governing Vessels [Motoyama, 1981].

There are a few nadis that are very unique, such as two of the three that make up the Sushuma. The two unique nadis are Ida and Pingala, which spiral around the chakra column, penetrating each chakra. They are believed to help awaken chakras to their next state of health and performance (figure 35). The ida channels more physically based PE upward and the pingala channels more spiritually based PE downward (figure 36). Most kundalini teachings I am aware of say that awakened kundalini raises up the sushuma, while a few others I have found say it can also travel down it (pingala).

The third nadi is sometimes called Sushuma, which is superimposed on the chakra column.

Nadis have also been described as existing deeper within the body, helping to circulate and store PE within the physical body's psychic anatomy that I call the Internal Aura. There are internal meridian descriptions as well, but they are less common. (The internal aura can be considered the field of collective consciousness of all your organs, cells and molecules. I do not teach it in this book for simplicity. Please see *The Psychic Anatomy Exercises* for more information and exercises involving it.)

Some deeper nadis mirror the pathway of meridians and vessels, potentially acting as a relay-amplifier for, or an antenna to, the PE these meridians and vessel radiate. It is probably these nadis that authors have described as internal meridians.

My experiences with these internal nadis have been very clear on a few occasions, especially one. The most significant is when I became aware of one that appeared to mirror my Lung Meridian (figure 28). It appeared expanded to be about four times wider and changed its pathway threw some muscles in my chest and shoulder after having a powerful back bending asana practice. When it changed its pathway, it appeared to approach a resistance when passing a group of muscle fibers. Eventually it snapped into place on the other side. This happened a few times as I moved before it stabilized and I lost awareness of it.

The changing of its pathway makes sense to me, because these streams of PE create electromagnetic fields and as they expand and body properties change, they need to move to find pathways of lower resistance[44].

You might be familiar with acupuncture, acupressure and/or other meridian therapies that use meridian points. There is a lot of potential in this complex subject for enhancing health and performance, but it is not something I discuss in this book, because of its complexity[45].

---

[44] If you like this topic, you might like *The Interface Between Psychic Energies and the Physical Body* and some of the chapters and appendices in *The Psychic Energy Reality.*

[45] In *The Psychic Anatomy Exercises* and *The Psychic Energy Reality* I give an overview of meridian points and some techniques for working with them.

Vessels Descriptions (Extraordinary Vessels)

Yang & Yin Heel Vessels and Yang & Yin Linking Vessels: These four vessels draw Earth PE from the ground and raise it up to the rest of the body and meridian system. My experiences have found these vessels powerful taps for vitality, providing strength and support to my physical body. The Yang ones draw upon more masculine type PE and the Yin more feminine types.

Griddle Vessel: This is a unique vessel that I have not had much experience with. It wraps around the waist, playing a role in the meridians and vessels that cross it and the surrounding anatomy. PE seem to circulate around it in both directions, helping to hold meridians and vessel in place. It is common to hear Traditional Chinese Medicine doctors comment on it being too tight or too loose.

Penetrating Vessel: Circulates male and female PE in the lower abdomen to send up the Conception and Governing Vessels when needed. I believe this vessel also helps to charge the tan tien. Its geometry and my experiences imply my description to be correct. It is possible that the Penetrating Vessel plays an important role in kundalini experiences as well. In regards to the experiences described as a raising of intense PE up the spine from the tail bone.

Governing Vessel: A more powerful meridian that draws in and radiates masculine PE to the entire meridian system and physical body.

Conception Vessel: A more powerful meridian that draws in and radiates feminine PE to the entire meridian system and physical body.

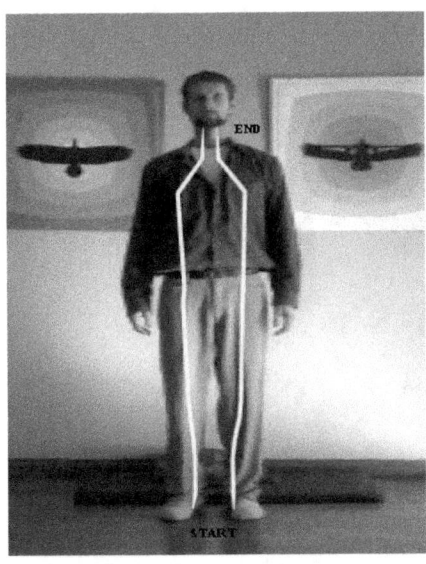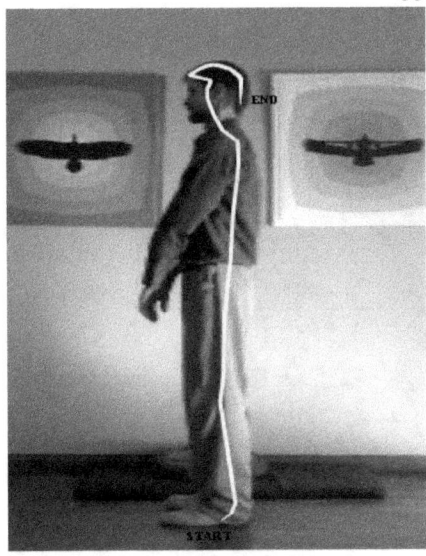

Figure 21: Yin Linking Vessel is shown on the left ad Yang Linking Vessel on the right.

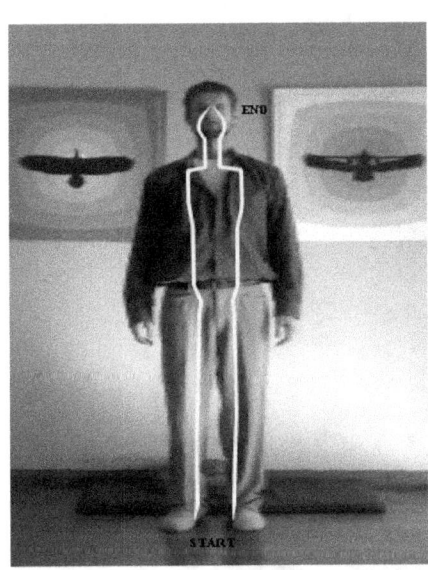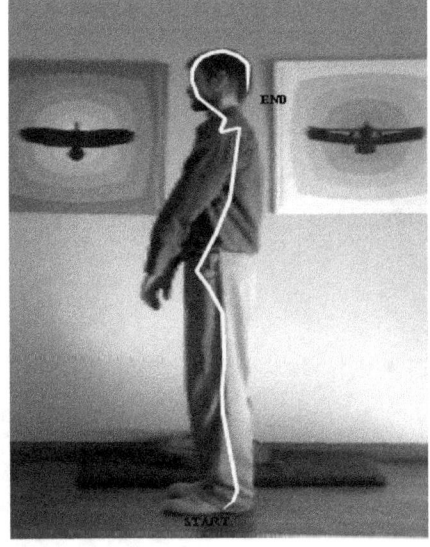

Figure 22: Yin Heel Vessel shown on the left and Yang Heel Vessel on the right.

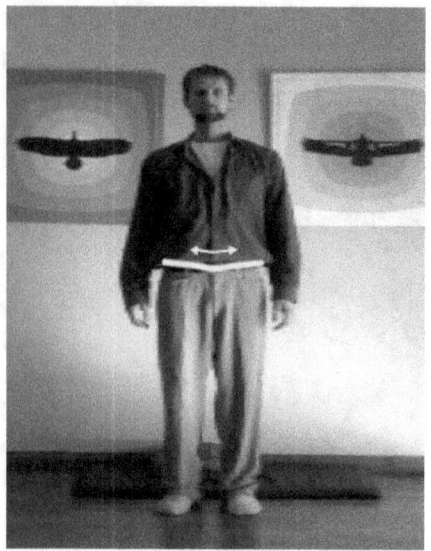
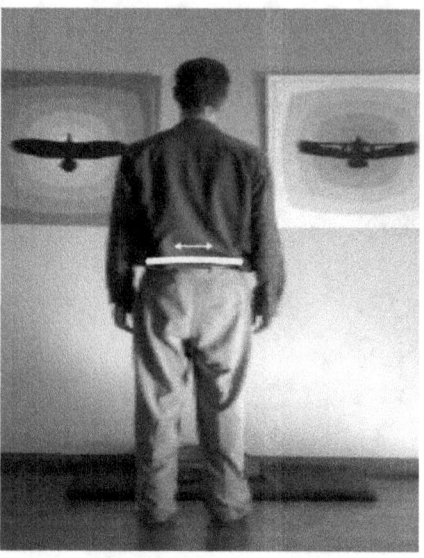

Figure 23: Griddle Vessel front view on left and back view on right.

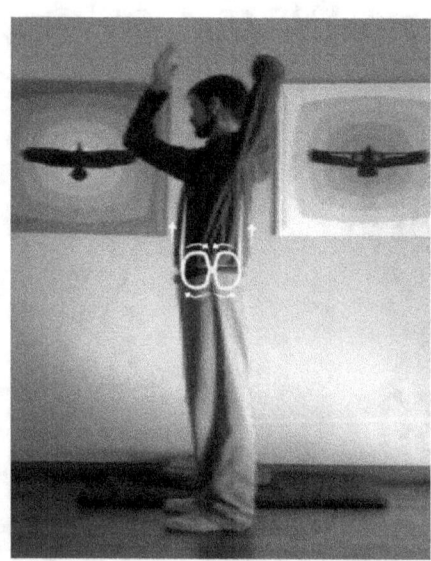

Figure 24: The Penetrating Vessel. You can see how it penetrates the center of the tan tien and is capable of shooting PE up the Governing and Conception Vessel (figures below), in a similar way to kundalini rising

descriptions.

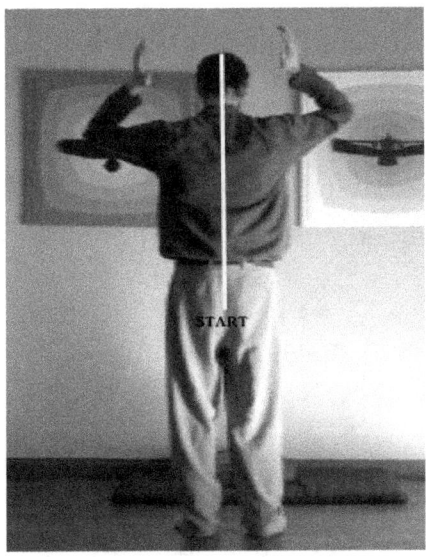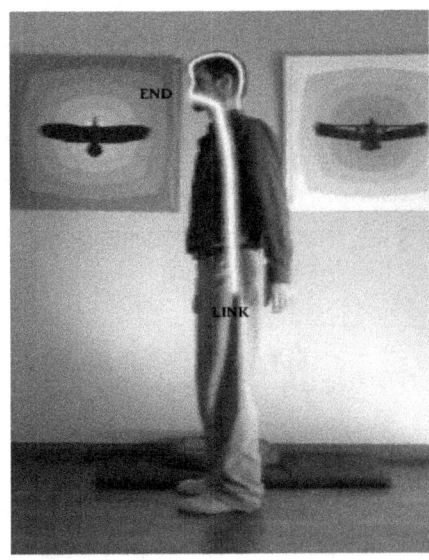

Figure 25: The Governing Vessel

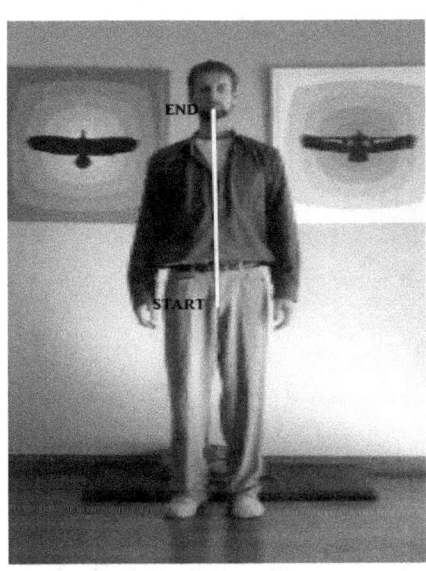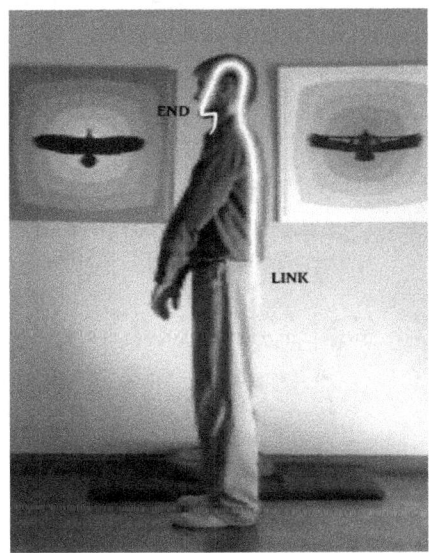

Figure 26: The Conception Vessel

Meridian Descriptions

Stomach Meridian: Draws in and radiates Earth-type PE inside the physical body from a masculine (yang) perspective[46] *to immediate physical structures and hollographically to those at a distance* (this comment in italic will not be repeated for each description). Food can considered a form of Earth.

Spleen Meridian: Draws in and radiates Earth-type PE inside the physical body from a feminine (yin) perspective[47].

Lung Meridian: Draws in and radiates Air-type PE inside the physical body from a masculine perspective. Lungs take in air.

Large Intestine Meridian: Draws in and radiates Air-type PE inside the physical body from a feminine perspective.

Kidney Meridian: Draws in and radiates Fire-type PE inside the physical body from a masculine perspective. Kidney meridian has always been associated with primal energies and action, which fire is associated with.

Bladder Meridian: Draws in and radiates Fire-type PE inside the physical body from a feminine perspective. Bladder meridian is commonly associated with feeding the major organs from the spine. The organs are always in a state of action

---

[46] A masculine perspective would be more of a left brained approach in both the type of PE drawn in and how they are radiated out within the physical body.

[47] A feminine perspective would be more of a right brained approach in both the type of PE drawn in and how they are radiated within the physical body.

(fire), building, dismantling and moving molecules.

Heart Meridian: Draws in and radiates Earth, Water, Air, Fire–type PE to balance and harmonize meridian activity from a masculine perspective. Heart meridian has always been associated with regulating the activity of the meridian system, hence it needs to work with all elemental forms of PE.

Small Intestine Meridian: Draws in and radiates Earth, Water, Air, Fire-type PE to balance and harmonize the meridian activity from a feminine perspective.

Gall Bladder: Draws in and radiates Water-type PE inside the physical body from a masculine perspective. Gall bladder meridian can be associated with going with the flow, as water goes with the flow.

Liver Meridian: Draws in and radiates Water-type PE inside the physical body from a feminine perspective. Liver meridian has been associated with anger, which is the emotion commonly experienced when things do not flow as we would like them to flow.

Pericardium Meridian: Draws in and radiates Earth, Water, Air, Fire-type PE to support meridian system to move PE to the chakras and/or parts of the body during times of stress from a feminine perspective. Supporting the activity of the meridian system is a common description for this meridian, hence it needs to work with all elemental PE.

Triple Heater: Draws in and radiates Earth, Water, Air, Fire-type PE to support the meridian system to move PE to the chakras and/or parts of the body during times of stress from a masculine perspective. Common teachings state that this meridian distributes PE to three burning spaces (heart, solar plexus and lower abdomen), which are very likely to be the fourth, third and second charkas based on their locations. I am not sure why these teachings do not include the first chakra. It is also common to see this meridian associated with the immune system and stress states in general.

I believe that all elemental PE are necessary in all meridians, but some of them work with specific ones more closely.

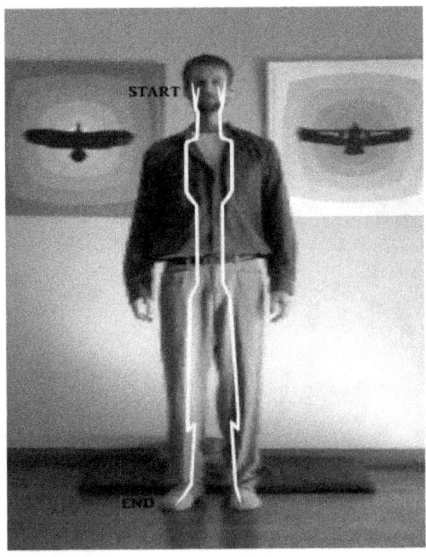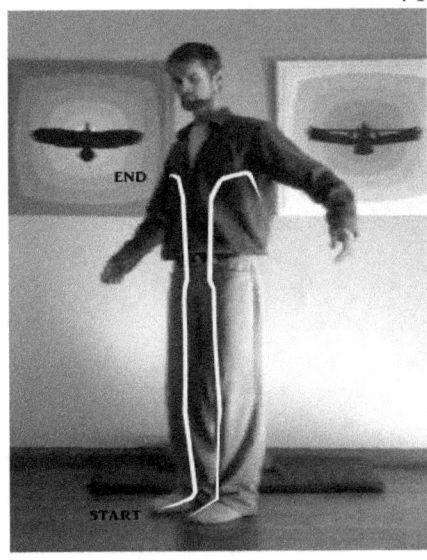

Figure 27: The Stomach Meridian (left). The Spleen Meridian (right). These meridians are paired.

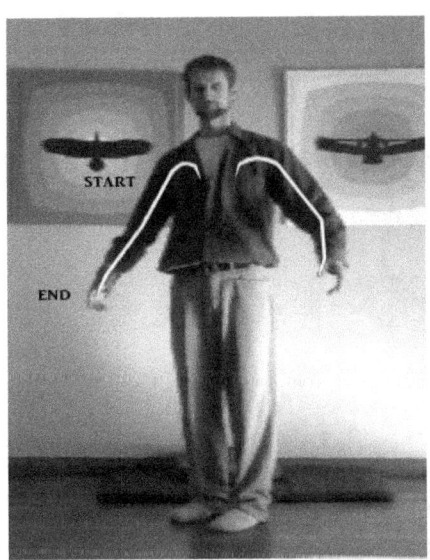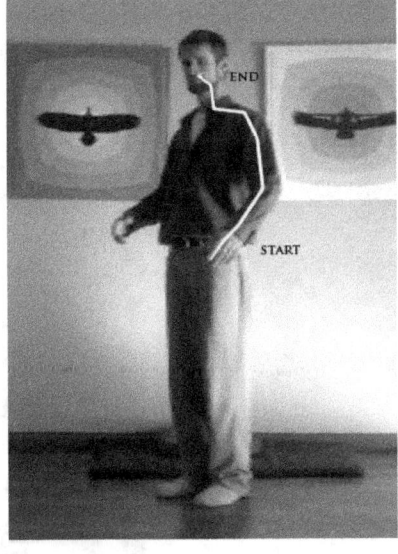

Figure 28: The Lung Meridian (left). The Large Intestine Meridian (right). It approaches the nose and then quickly shots back towards the ear. These meridians are paired.

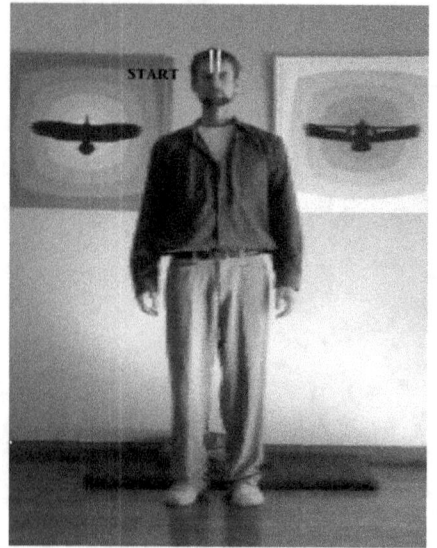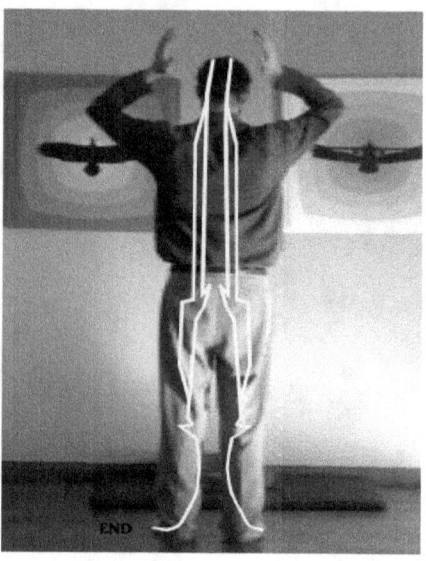

Figure 29: The Bladder Meridian. Paired with the Kidney Meridian.

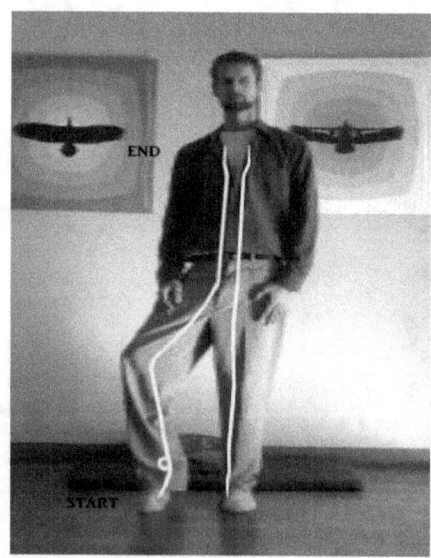

Figure 30: The Kidney Meridian. Curls around the heel. Paired with the
Bladder Meridian.

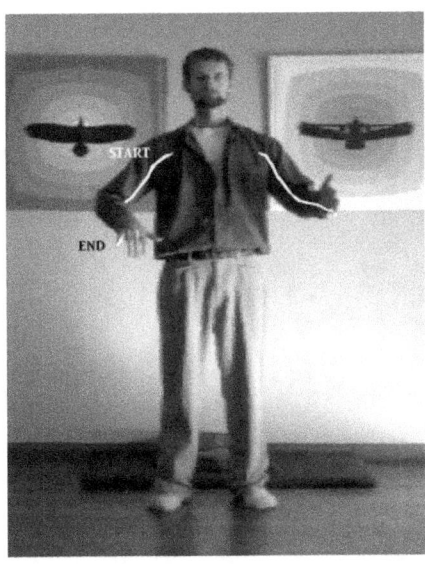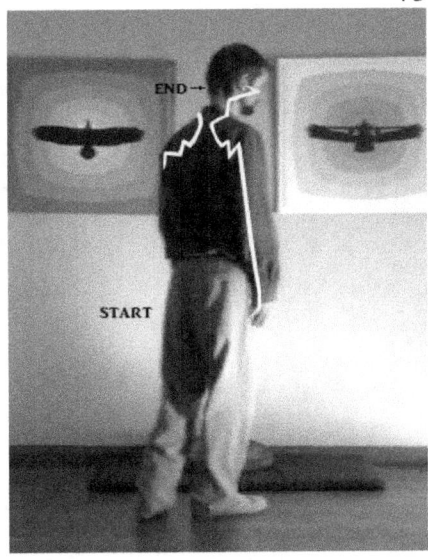

Figure 31: The Heart Meridian (left), curls from the inside of the palm to the end of the pinky finger. The Small Intestine Meridian (right), shots towards the ear when it gets to the corner of the eye. These meridians are paired.

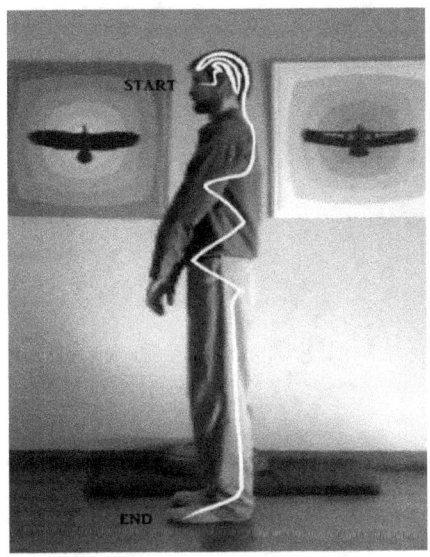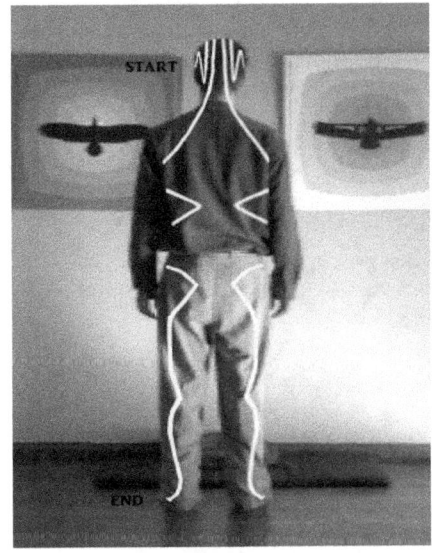

Figure 32: The Gall Bladder Meridian. Paired with the Liver Meridian.

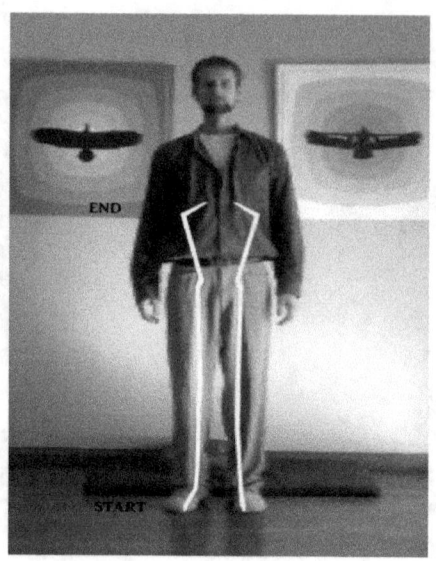

Figure 33: The Liver Meridian. Paired with the Gall Bladder Meridian.

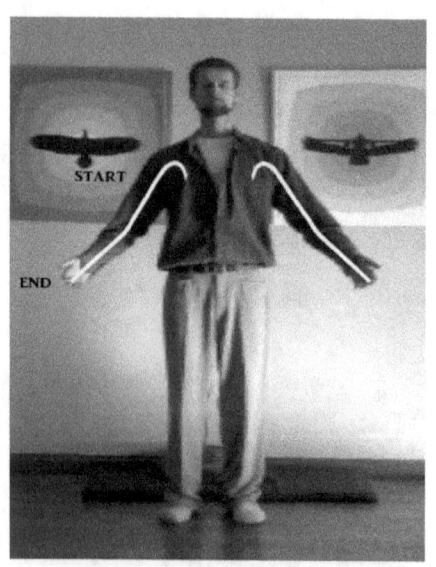
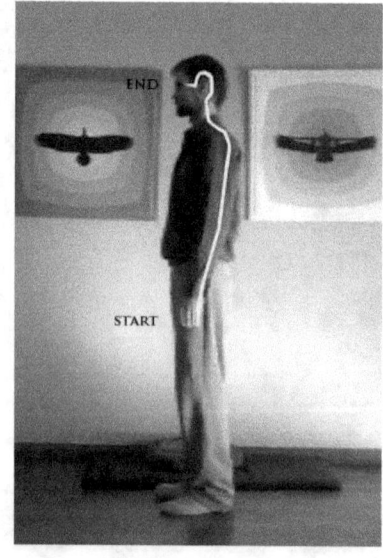

Figure 34: The Paracadium Meridian (left). The Triple Heater Meridian
(right). These meridians are paired.

As you develop the health and performance of your aura, your meridians will naturally start increasing in theirs as well. This can be facilitated by tracing healthy PE threw them. Tracing healthy PE threw your meridians is great for expanding them to clear out unhealthy PE and fill them with healthy PE.

Meridians can be compared to veins and the aura as a muscle. You can work your aura/muscles hard to develop them, but your meridians/veins are better developed as a consequence of your developing aura/muscles. So when working with your meridians, just make sure they are healthy, balanced and harmonized using a moderate amount of focus (intense focus makes PE more powerful).

Working with the meridians and vessels can be complicated to learn, but well worth it, especially in the beginning. If it is too much to do at once, I recommend periodically looking at the meridian figures and tracing them. Even if it is just one or two meridians or vessels a day, it will make it easier to get good at the exercises in time.

Vessel Exercise 1

Tracing healthy PE threw your vessels can be very rewarding. Follow the sequence and pathways shown in the figures, focusing on the healthiest PE for each one when tracing them with your tip finger tips or palms.

When changing between the first four vessels, move directly to the next start point. In Level 5 of my book *The Psychic Anatomy Exercises,* I share a routine that incorporates physical body systems, which makes the changes between these vessels more purposeful.

The griddle and thrusting vessels are different to trace. I recommend Holding PE and awareness of them with the intent of enhancing their health and performance, moving your hands intuitively when guided. Be mindful of the tension your griddle vessel places on your meridians. There is an optimal tension for every moment, which you will learn with practice.

Circulating PE in the thrusting vessel can be visualized and even traced by swirling your hands by your sides in the directions of flow. I like to do this while giving attention to my conception and governing vessels. I find it helps harmonize and balance these three vessels as well as empower them. Sometimes the thrusting vessel will seem to be feeding the conception and governing vessels more than at other times.

When you are done move onto Vessel Exercise 2.

Vessel Exercise 2

It is commonly taught that pressing your tongue to the top of your mouth helps improve the connection between the conception and governing vessels. Do this and start tracing a healthy balance of masculine and feminine PE down your throat, visualizing them washing threw your lungs, stomach and intestines. As you reach your anus, focus on releasing any unhealthy PE to the Earth and/or vegetation for recycling. In the beginning it is a good idea to repeatedly sweep threw your colon, because unhealthy PE tend to collect there.

At this point, shift your attention to the healthiest conception vessel energies (feminine PE) and sweep them up threw your conception vessel. At your mouth, shift your attention to the healthiest balance of feminine and masculine energies and trace them threw your sinuses, brain, down your spine and out your tail bone where they will connect with you governing vessel.

Shift your attention to the healthiest masculine energies and trace threw your governing vessel and when you get to your mouth, repeat the process.

These two vessels are much more commonly found in records regarding the Meridian System. A major and common difference in their description is that they have meridian points and the other vessels do not. This difference has resulted in some people calling the vessels in Vessel Exercise 1 the 6 Extraordinary Vessels and the governing and conception vessels, Vessels.

I have found that giving the governing and conception vessels more attention than the others is sometimes a good idea. For example, just tracing them and not the others during a practice session.

Ending your practice with extraordinary vessel charging is a good way to charge yourself up, fueling the changes your practice has helped initiate, and for grounding. As you advance with this exercise, you can incorporate connecting and drawing upon healthy Earth PE, especially into your heel and linking vessels. I have found this to be very grounding and empowering.

Meridian Exercise

When you are about done tracing your governing vessel (at the hair line), you can switch over to your stomach meridian. Focusing on the healthiest PE for it, follow it to the end and then switch over to your spleen meridian. Continue with this process in the order that the meridians are presented in the descriptions and figures, focusing on the healthiest PE for each one. As you do this, take note of any areas that might need more attention and return to them when you are done to trace again and apply other techniques; discussed below.

When you are done these exercises and have addressed the areas that caught your attention, stay in a meditative and intend for your meridians and vessels to be balanced and harmonized together.

You can also repeat these exercises, giving you the additional benefits for the same reasons as discussed at the end of Chakra Exercise 2.

Comments on Vessel and Meridian Exercises

As you trace vessels and meridians, you will eventually become aware of energy centers as you pass over them, such as your chakras and pockets of PE. If you feel you have found something that needs more attention, you can remember it down for later or work on them as you find them. Dealing with them in the moment can be distracting and they might deal with themselves as you continue with your practice. Be intuitive and be biased towards not working with them right away.

When working with them, you have the option of Holding a field of healthy PE around them and/or applying other General Techniques. These areas can and often have inner issues associated with them[48]. You will become more aware of their nature as you work with them.

When trying to work with these areas and you have already done both the vessel and meridian exercises, you can repeatedly trace the meridian associated with the area (if there is one) and sometimes it is a good idea to repeatedly trace the meridian it is paired with as well. Other techniques that can help are discussed in regards to working with pockets of PE

---

[48] Inner issues are also know as core beliefs of unhealthy patterns. Discussed in *Inner and Outer Success.*

below.

Nadi Exercise

Just intending and visualizing nadis inside of your body and the inside of your body in general glowing and being healthy can help empower them. This concept can be used when focusing on balancing and harmonizing your vessels and meridians as discussed above. You can also include your aura in this[49].

Sushuma Exercise

Just focusing on ida and pingala being active/powering up with your central nadi can be a rewarding experience as well (figures 35 & 36). Especially when you include your chakra column and chakras. This approach is more effective for awakening purposes, because it can be held for a longer period of time, allowing balance and harmony to be maintained as power increases naturally or intentionally. Pulsing PE threw them as discussed after the figures combines very well with asanas.

---

[49] This is a concept associated with doing a General Alignment. General Alignments discussed in Chapter 11.

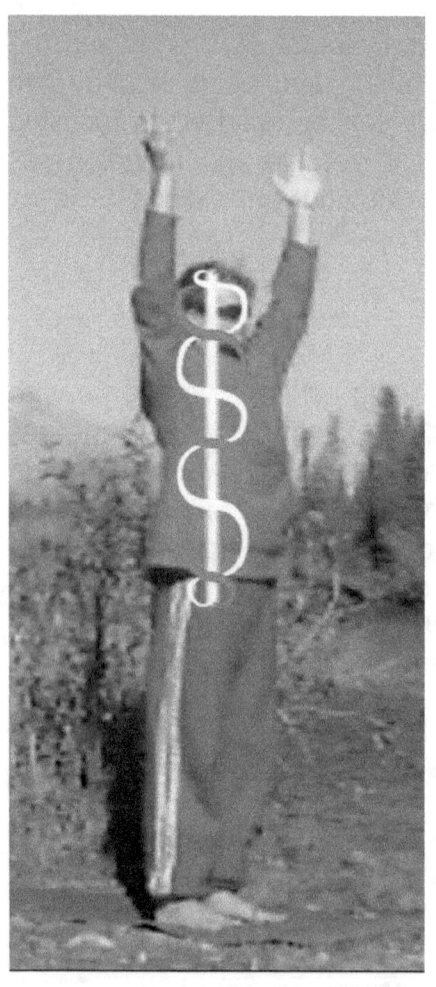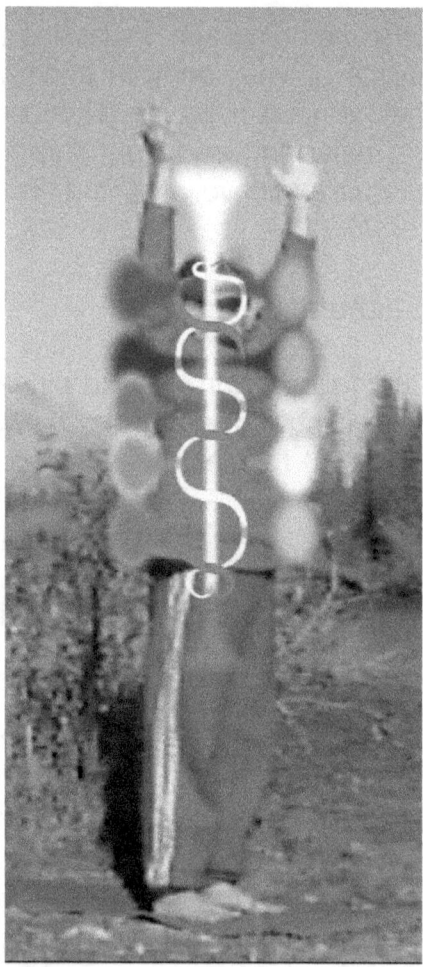

Figure 35: On the left is just the Sushuma and on the right the Chakras are included as well. You can see how ida and pingala penetrate each chakra.

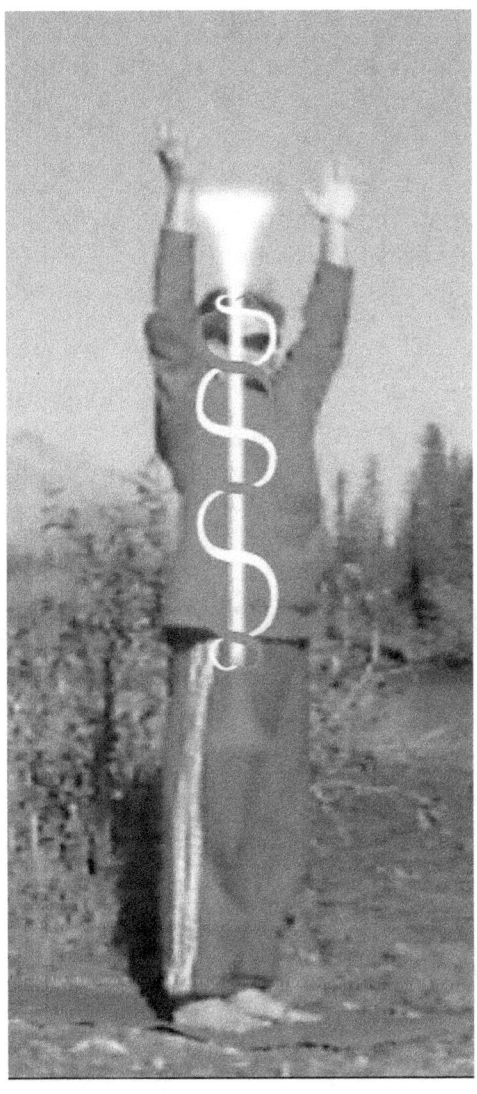

Figure 36: I included this image to give you the visual of how your pingala (white) and ida (red) are connected to your seventh (white) and first chakras (red).

This exercise mimics and can stimulate kundalini experiences. Many teachings say to let kundalini out the top of your head (seventh chakra), but I encourage you to learn to release it more slowly and keep it circulating in your sushuma to get as much benefit from it as possible. Earth kundalini will spiral up ida and then travel down your central nadi (chakra column) and Heaven kundalini will spiral down pingala and up your central nadi. When they power up as described above, a very physical part of your psychic anatomy is empowered, creating a foundation for great things to happen.

> Remember, too much power without sufficient balance and harmony can be a hindrance to your development and uncomfortable to your psyche in all psychic energy practices, especially this one.

I like to send a pulse threw ida and my psychic anatomy general when moving from Forward Fold to Standing. Often I will combine this with Conducting/Embracing Earth. Once standing, I like to Conduct/Embrace Heaven down pingala and my psychic anatomy in general. When returning back to Forward Fold, I like to send a clearing Sweep (pulse) down pingala and my psychic anatomy in general as well sometimes.

Meridian Mudra

Meridian Mudra helps connect meridian pairs (see Meridian Descriptions above) at the hands. I recommend using this mudra to help balance and harmonize your meridian system.

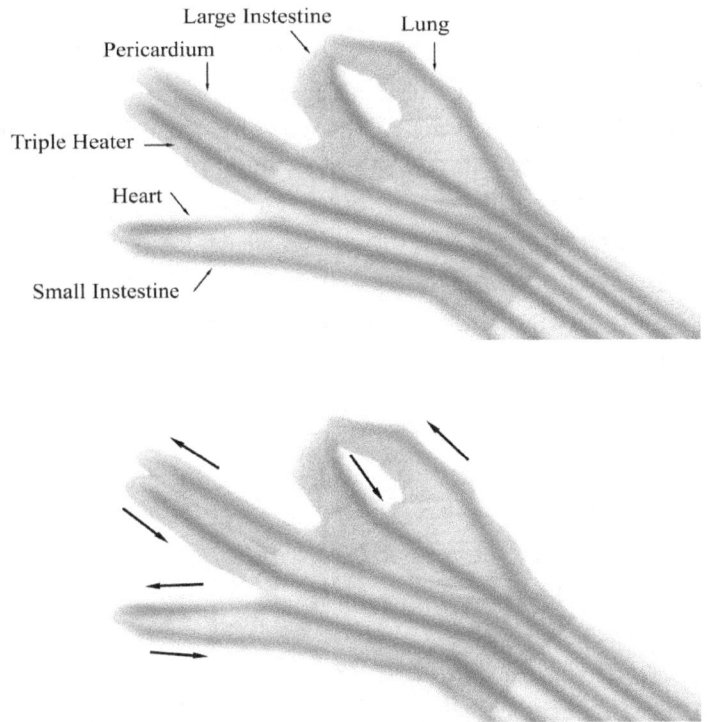

Figure 37: Meridian Mudra. Bottom image shows the direction PE flow. Blue means the meridian is on the other side of the hand.

Combining Aura and Meridian Exercises

It is usually best to start with the aura exercises and then do the meridian exercises above, because the aura exercises cultivate large amounts of healthy PE that the meridian exercises make use of. Cycling between them is best, because as unhealthy PE are released from one of them, associated PE can be released more easily in the other. The same is true for integrating healthy PE associated with our development. This can be done for specific virtues as well as in general; discussed below. These two comments hold true for all Psychic Anatomy Exercises. Cycling is a very powerful concept!

Working with Pockets of Unhealthy Psychic Energies

When you find areas that need attention during these exercises, the common response is to focus healthy PE into and around them. This form of healing works well in most cases, but if you keep coming back to the same areas over time, it would be wise to focus your attention on finding any inner issues that might be associated with them[50]. Doing this will make it easier for them to release. I recommend *Inner and Outer Success* for the best of conventional self-help and many psychic energy based techniques.

I recommend the following authors for insights on correlations between body parts and mental/emotional inner issues that could be associated with these pockets, as well as other physical conditions. This is a developing science, so get a few opinions.

Louise Hay, You *can Heal our Life*
Karol Truman, *Feelings Buried Alive Never Die*
Carolyn Mein, *Releasing Emotional Patterns with Essential Oils*
Traditional Chinese Medicine books
Ayurvedic Medicine books

More on working with pocket of psychic energies in Chapter 8.

---

[50] Inner issues are be unhealthy belief patterns. Discussed in depth within *Inner and Outer Success.*

Meditation and Grounding Comments

Practice these exercises well and remember to stay in meditation afterward to focus on being balanced and harmonized. During these meditations, visions, insights and facilitation from your spirit guides/angels can happen. Remember to always do Grounding after these exercises as well, and during when it feels appropriate. Being grounded is important for living to your fullest potential.

Practicing these exercises will develop your awareness of the parts of your psychic anatomy so far discussed. Once you have a few experiences with these exercises and feel the parts of your psychic anatomy so far discussed are in a good state of health and performance, you are ready to move onto the next Chapter.

There are more meridian exercises, as well as psychic anatomy exercises in general within *The Psychic Anatomy Exercises* that can help you achieve greater states of health and performance. The ones in this book are just the essentials.

CHAPTER 6
YOUR HARA

Your Hara is a very significant part of your psychic anatomy. Compared to your aura and meridians, your hara is made up of PE closer to those associated with your soul. It holds patterns of energy that influence the way your aura forms, helping to shape your interests and desires to move you in the direction of your life's purpose/destiny.

Recall that PE, especially those in your psychic anatomy and specifically in your aura, influence you to experience the emotions and thoughts associated with them. When your hara empowers or oppresses certain PE in your psychic anatomy, it shapes you to have specific interests and desires.

External influences can over-power a person's hara, especially if they are strong and/or their hara is weak. This is seen in modern societies as people strive towards the norm, only to feel discontent with what they have achieved later in life. Modern society poses many powerful influences. Hence, it is important to have a strong and health hara. Many successful people have a healthy and strong hara system[51]. The hara exercises below and Psychic Anatomy Exercises in general can help empower your hara.

The hara has three centers and a vertical column called the hara line that connects them together and the hara in general to the Earth (see figure 38). Some of your best Psychic Anatomy Yoga postures will come from aligning your spine with your hara line as your balance is being challenged. Focusing on your hara line's connection to the Earth as you do this can greatly help

---

[51] Brennan, 1993 discusses this as well.

empower your psychic anatomy with Earth PE, helping you be more grounded and in control. This concept is discussed again in the Heaven and Earth Exercises below.

The Tan Tein (also known as the lower tan tien) is a popular center in Asian cultures and best known for being taught in martial arts. It is believed to be a power-center that stores PE to help empower the psychic energy memories in your aura that are in harmony with how your hara. Another way to word this is that it helps empower the psychic energy memories that keep you living your life's purpose/destiny.

The Soul Seat (also known as the middle tan tien) plays a more active role in helping to shape the way psychic energy memories form in your aura. It is similar to how your tan tein functions, but is more focused on changing psychic energy memories than empowering them. For example, the PE associated with being interested in a sport, such as hockey can be reshaped to being interested in the physical health and performance of the athletes, which can be reshaped further to being interested in many things outside of hockey, such as your own physical health and performance.

If the influences of drinking, socializing and/or belonging/acceptance over-power are dominant in your interest of hockey, it is more difficult for your soul seat to reshape your interests to guide you along such a path. There are many examples like this. It is always wise to check in with yourself and maybe get some space to make sure you are not investing your time for such reasons[52].

---

[52] See *Inner and Outer Success* for details.

The Soul Gate[53] is a center above your head (see figure 38). It helps connect you more directly to our soul. Usually this center shines the PE of virtues upon you (figure 40), but also sends PE to help reshape your soul seat and psychic anatomy in general. As your soul/you evolve in this life and from past lives, virtues are learned and your soul gate develops a connection to very fundamental and pure forms of PE associated with virtues, popularly called called Rays[54].

It is also very common for your soul gate to send PE to your seventh chakra, which is often experienced as mental intuition, invention, innovation, general creativity and/or the channeling your higher-self. By developing the health and performance of your psychic anatomy, these skills get easier to use, which makes it easier to use them more often, as well as for these center to focus their powers in others ways as well. Such as manifesting your future.

There are believed to be additional soul gates above the one in figure 40; see figure 46. These centers have also been called the chakras above the head by several authors. The next one up connects you to your soul's soul, which is called your over soul, the next to your second over-soul and so on all the way back to the omnipresent state many spiritual and religious teachers talk about (God).

You can work with your hara the same way you work with your aura. Focus on empowering each hara center with the healthiest PE for it. After completing all centers, focus on balancing and harmonizing all of them individually and together.

---

[53]   There are upper soul gates as well. Discussed in *The Psychic Anatomy Exercises* and *The Psychic Energy Reality.*

[54]   Common in Ascended Master Teachings and Hinduism.

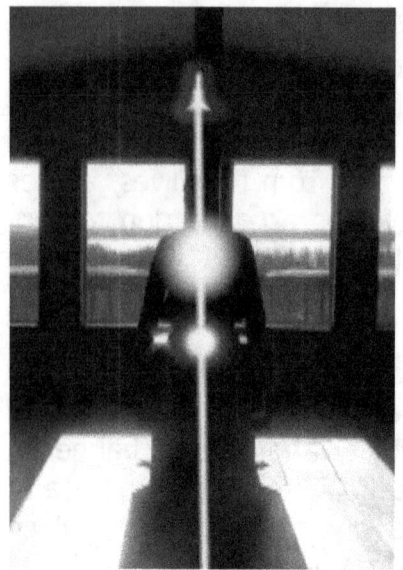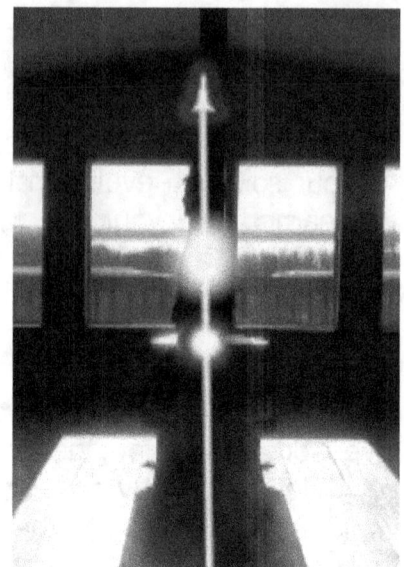

Figure 38: Shows the front view of the Human Hara on the left and a side view on the right. Only the first soul gate is shown

Hara Exercise

Start by focusing on connecting your hara line deep within the Earth. Then bringing your hands down to your sides, directing your palms to face the Earth and your hara line as you focus on empowering your hara line with healthy Earth PE. After for five-ten breaths, move your hands to face your tan tien, focusing healthy PE for it as you Hold, Pulsate or use other General Techniques.

Once you feel you have spent enough time at your tan tein (five-ten breaths recommended), float your hands up towards your soul seat and empower it with the healthiest PE for it in the same way. When you feel you have spent enough time with it, float your hands up to face your first soul gate, empowering it in the same way as well.

If you feel drawn to work with your upper soul gates, you can progress to them after your first is done. If not, just leave them out of your practice until you do. It could take several months of practice before they feel right to work with. A good foundation is needed first, so be patient.

When you feel you are done, spend some time focusing on these centers being balanced and harmonized individually and together.

Its optional to focus on your hara line pulling your spine straight. Letting your knees slightly bend and your tail bone curve under to help straighten your spine to align with your hara line. This posture can help ground you to the Earth, empowering your hara and entire being in general. This is often taught in qi-gong and martial arts for these reasons.

Although simple, this exercise can take you into deep states of meditation and strongly trigger your intuitive guidance; especially with practice. It can be very challenging do anything physical and maintain deep meditative states, so keep a pen and paper near by to record insights as the exercises progress and especially for afterward, before your insights fade away like dreams[55].

Tan Tien Exercise

Your tan tien provides strength to psychic energy memories in your psychic anatomy. When practicing Psychic Anatomy Yoga, changes that occur in your psychic anatomy will likely affect your tan tien on all its levels as old patterns are broken down and new ones established. You can charge your tan tien with PE that support these changes after your practice. Lots of these PE will come from within the Earth. This will speed up your

---

[55] Their nature is very similar.

92
progress.

Addressing these changes as they are happening by including the intent of charging your tan tien with supportive PE can be done as well. For example, when you are charging a part(s) of your psychic anatomy to enhance their health and performance, you can include your tan tien with the intent of releasing and empowering the patterns that are associated with the area(s).

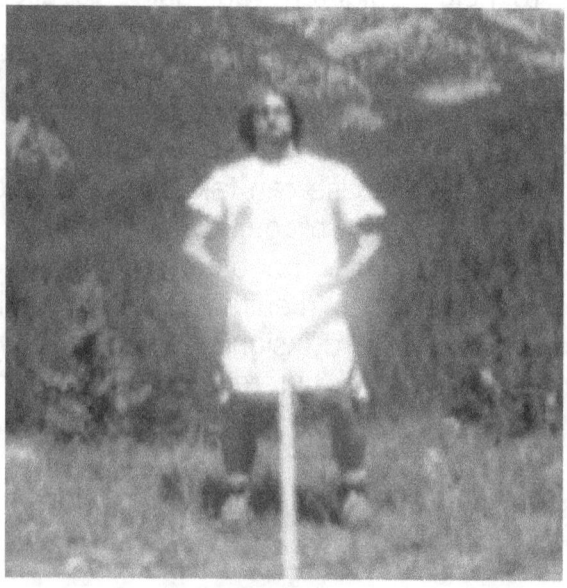

Figure 39: Shows tan tien connecting to the Earth, helping to empower healthy PE and psychic energies within the psychic anatomy.

Sine Wave

Sine Wave is very similar to the Yin-Yang posture, but your finger tips of your hand at the bottom of your reach face down your hara line towards the Earth and your other hand's finger tips point up your hara line towards your soul gates. Sine Wave is used to help balance, harmonize and align your hara system.

From Sine Wave you can also float your hands up and down in front of you, circulating PE as Scanning. You may feel guided to let your hands move to specific hara centers as you do this, giving them more attention. Trust your intuition.

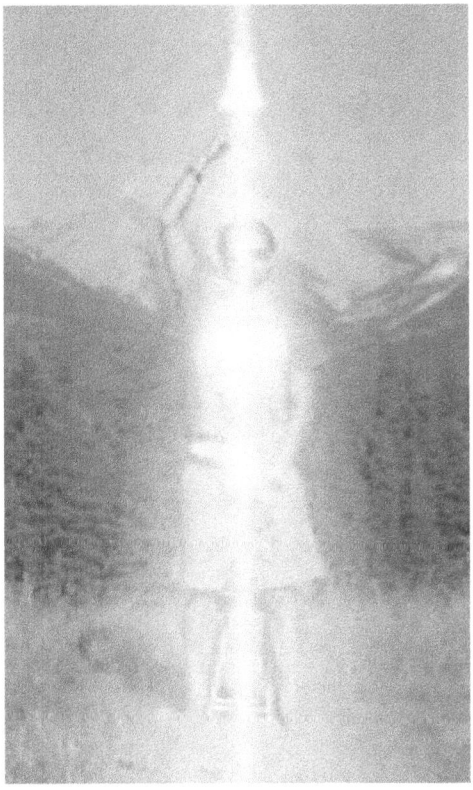

Figure 40: Shows Sine Wave, as well as the first Soul Gate shining PE.

CHAPTER 7
YOUR CORE STAR

When your aura, meridians and hara are in a good state of health and performance, you have a good foundation for empowering your Core Star. Your core star is believed to be the part of your soul that has incarnated. It can expand and contract to empower your hara when needed and even your aura. As you do the core star exercise below, your core star can feed from your soul gates as well, building power that will help empower how it influences your psychic anatomy.

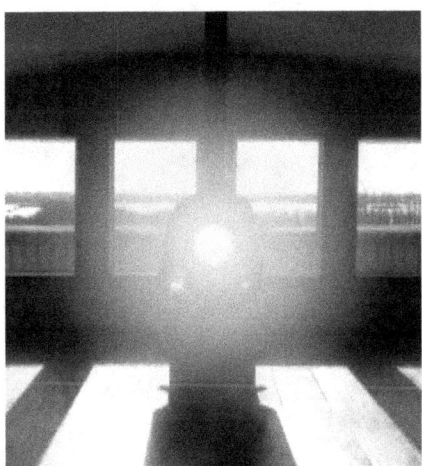 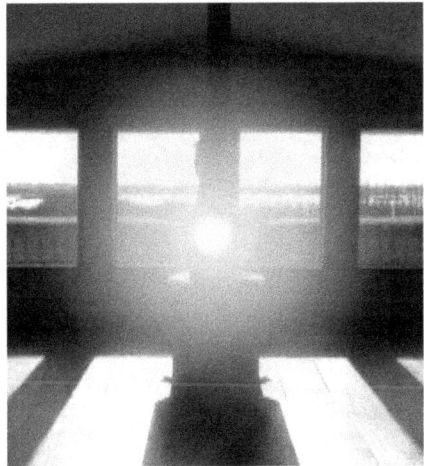

Figure 41: Shows the front view of the Human Core Star on the left and a side view on the right.

Core Star Exercise

With your aura, meridians and hara charged with healthy PE, balanced and harmonized (do this first with previous exercises), turn your attention to your core star, moving your palms to face it. This exercise is extremely simple, but a lot can happen during it. Intuitive Movements can be more common here as the empowerment of your core star can influence changes to occur almost any where in your psychic anatomy.

When you feel you have spent enough time empowering and connecting to your core star, spend some time focusing on it and your psychic anatomy in general being balanced and harmonized.

98

CHAPTER 8
WORKING WITH POCKETS OF PSYCHIC ENERGIES

The information below can come in handy at almost anytime while practicing the psychic energy exercises in this book. They will most often be used as unhealthy and healthy pockets of PE are found while Scanning.

Working with Pockets of Unhealthy Psychic Energies

Pockets of unhealthy PE usually feel dark and congested; basically unhealthy. When finding them, which can be anywhere in your psychic anatomy. The common response is to ignore them and let your practice take care of them, returning to them later to make sure they have been dealt with or working with them directly.

In general, working with them directly is best done after giving your practice, because changes in seemingly unrelated areas could make a big difference to releasing them. When you are working with them directly, focus healthy PE upon them using the General Techniques. This will work well in most cases, but not always.

Unhealthy pockets of PE can resist your efforts, which is sometimes the consequence of them being connected to other pockets in other parts of you. For example, if you become aware of a pocket of unhealthy PE in your shoulder that is not releasing easily, try focusing on becoming aware of any areas (and inner issues[56]) associated with it. Such an association might be in your aura, hara, physical body, or with an emotion

---

[56] Discussed below.

or thought. Every part of you is interconnected. This is the mind-body-spirit connection.

This will work well in most cases, but if you keep coming back to the same area(s) over time and/or have lingering unhealthy emotions and/or thoughts, it would be wise to focus your attention on finding any psychological issues (aka. inner issues) associated with it. This is best done with in Experiential Meditation with the intent to become aware of associated inner issues and/or using psychological/self-help technique(s)[57].

Psychological/self-help techniques can be very effective in these situations and compliment the surfacing of them as well. I recommend learning some psychological/self-help techniques to compliment your efforts with Psychic Anatomy Yoga. As you empower yourself with healthy PE, inner issues will be pushed to the surface as a form of detoxifying them. These techniques can greatly facilitate the process, making it easier. I discuss the best of self-help techniques and some newer ones based more in PE within *Inner and Outer Success.*

It is common for deep exhalations to occur when unhealthy PE are released. The famous Fire Breathing technique, which uses rapid inhalations and exhalations, often associated with kundalini experiences, can be very useful to facilitate such releases. If you are mindful of using Fire Breathing for this purpose, it will happen naturally more easily.

Working with Pockets of Healthy Psychic Energies

Pockets of healthy PE usually feel bright and expanded; basically healthy. When you find these pockets, you can ignore them and let your practice help to empower and integrate them

---

[57] For the best of conventional self-help and many psychic energy techniques, see *Inner and Outer Success.*

into your psychic anatomy naturally or focus on finding associated areas that you can work with to help empower and integrate them. Usually this is best done near the end of your practice to allow for seemingly unrelated changes to occur in other parts of yourself, making the process easier.

Sometimes these associated areas will be pockets of unhealthy PE that need to be released or just parts of your psychic anatomy that need to be prepared. For example, expanding the heart/fourth charka to make it easier to connect to the PE associated with the healthy pocket. Here's another example. You become aware of a healthy pocket in or near your heart/fourth chakra and when focusing on associated areas become aware of unhealthy PE in your sacral/2nd chakra that need to be released to allow your heart/fourth to embrace the change. This could mean that your heart/fourth chakra is enhancing its abilities to form relationships, but there is an emotion that hinders it. Recall that your fourth chakra works with the PE of relationships and your 2nd chakra with the PE of emotions.

These pockets are often associated with the development of virtues and/or skills. You can facilitate them by practicing the Psychic Anatomy Yoga with the intent of developing the virtues and/or skills in a general/specific way[58]. Remember, the more specific you are, the more power your intentions will have[59]. Try starting with a general intention and mindfully getting more specific.

As you learn to work with your inner issues as taught in my book *Inner and Outer Success,* you'll learn ways to identify which virtues are most important to you, making it easier to focus your attention more specifically in the ways just discussed.

---

[58] Remember to be intuitive. Sometimes we only think we know, but intuition will always know better.
[59] PE are controlled by your attention.

CHAPTER 9
FINAL COMMENTS

Improving the health and performance of your psychic anatomy is the main focus of Psychic Anatomy Yoga. As your psychic anatomy improves, it will work better independently and collectively, which will improve your psychic and physical health and performance.

There is enough information presented so far to keep you developing the health and performance of your psychic anatomy for years. The information in the next section can be added to your practice when you are ready. They will help empower, balance and harmonize your psychic anatomy in more masterful ways. Be patient before exploring them, because they rely on a good foundation in the psychic energy exercises already discussed.

If you are eager to incorporate the exercises already discussed into your asana practice, all of them can be done incorporated nicely whenever your find yourself into a standing position and even just with a vertical spine (ex. Warrior poses).

As you get better at doing these exercises, you'll become more aware of details and be able to empower yourself more specifically as you go through different stages of your life. Try devoting sessions of practice to specific virtues and/or skills. This will help empower the associated PE on all levels of your psychic anatomy, facilitating your development.

I recommend practicing with a group. The team-effort of a group pulls in an abundance of healthy PE (much more than the

104

sum of its parts) that are in general more harmonized[60]. The group also pulls in a more diverse spectrum of PE that the whole group can benefit from. This diversity is a result of some people being more developed in some ways than others. We are all different. Group practice is discussed in Appendix A.

As you get more powerful with these exercises, you will have more profound experiences and faster results. The exercises in the next section will help you get these results more easily.

---

[60] If there are too many disharmonious people in a group and the group doesn't know how to create and sustain harmony, this statement is not true.

106

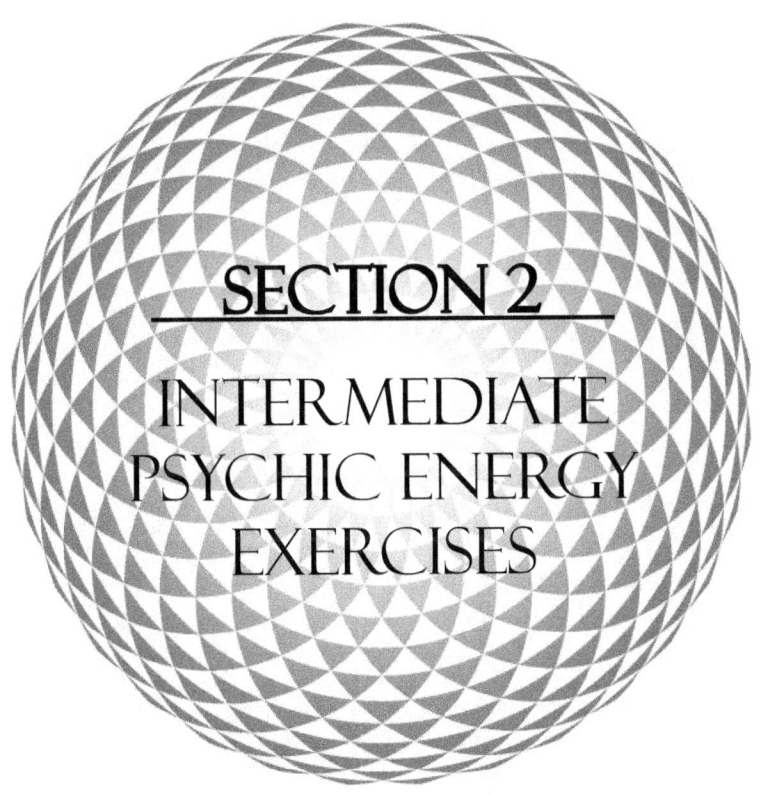

SECTION 2

INTERMEDIATE PSYCHIC ENERGY EXERCISES

CHAPTER 10
HEAVEN AND EARTH EXERCISES

These exercises make use of the psychic anatomy of planet Earth. The PE of Heaven come from above your head, sometimes way above your head where PE are less complex[61] and more spiritual in nature. The PE of Earth come from within the Earth, which are also less complex[62], but of a more physical nature (life force) than spiritual. Drawing these energies into and threw your being (body and psychic anatomy) is the purpose of the Heaven and Earth Exercises.

You at consider Earth energies more dense and rigid and heaven energies more lite and plastic. The lite and plastic qualities allow for specific patterns of PE to be formed, while the dense and rigid qualities make it easier for these patterns to sustain themselves in the complex psychic energy environment on the Earth's surface.

When I use the word Embracing, it refers to just incubating yourself with one of these energies, while Conducting refers to channel them threw you into the other. For example, Embracing Heaven would have you connecting to and incubating yourself with the PE of heaven that help you live to your fullest potential. Conducting Heaven would have you channeling the PE of heaven into the Earth. Both have their advantages.

Embracing Heaven is a more refined and sensitive process when it comes to integrating with these PE; this usually plays an important role in developing new psychic energy memories. Conducting Heaven can still help develop new psychic energy

---

[61] Most psychic energy complexity happens on the surface of Earth.
[62] Most psychic energy complexity happens on the surface of Earth.

memories (PE are still absorbed as when Embracing Heaven), but in a more powerful and less refined way. The power of this flow of PE also makes Conducting Heaven more cleansing. Another advantage is that once the conducted PE resonant with the PE within the Earth, they become more stable and easier to integrate within yourself. Its a balance between power (Conducting) and refinement (Embracing), which usually happens naturally/intuitively.

Advantages and disadvantages of Embracing Earth are similar to Embracing Heaven. Embracing Earth can be more refined and sensitive in regards to developing new psychic energy memories. Conducting Earth helps develop new psychic energy memor and other treatments to help get ies in a more powerful and less refined way. It can also help create resonance between PE of Earth and PE of heaven, with the PE of heaven helping to refine the PE of Earth as they are drawn closer closer to the Earth's surface.

Especially Conducting can be demanding on your psychic anatomy, which is good, because it exercises it. Using the general technique of Scanning can help you find areas that hinder Conducting. (In general, the slower you Scan the more of a connection you will make with your psychic anatomy, which will help you find areas that need more attention.) Either these areas will be weak with unhealthy PE or depleted, needing empowerment with healthy PE. Pulsating, Pulsate Breathing, Sweeping and those discussed in Chapter 2 are common techniques for addressing these areas.

Sweeping your hands threw your psychic anatomy and/or over your physical body facilitates these currents of PE, helping unhealthy PE to be released and healthy PE to flow freely. Combining a deep-natural exhalation with a quicker Sweep can move lots of energy that has surfaced for release all at once. Using a quick Sweep near the end of a sweeping motion can help throw unhealthy PE away from you. When doing this, intend for the unhealthy energies to continue moving until they are completely released and on their way into the Earth and/or vegetation for recycling. Often, repeated Sweeps are needed to make sure an area is cleared well. There is a lot of freedom on how you use this technique. Sweep as much as you want until you feel the area(s) is sufficiently cleared.

There are eight different ways to do the Heaven and Earth Exercises. Just Embracing Heaven or just Embracing Earth, just Conducting Heaven or just Conducting Earth, Embracing Heaven and Earth, Conducting Heaven and Earth, Embracing Heaven/Earth and Conducting Earth/Heaven. When Heaven and Earth Exercises are mentioned below, I will be referring to any of these combinations. I've given a few examples of these exercises below.

When choosing which Heaven and Earth Exercise to use, there is only one thing I advise, be in the moment and intuitive.

Conducting/Embracing Heaven

Embracing Heaven is a popular technique in many qi-gong, martial practices, as well as religious practices[63]. It has also been taught under other names in different practices as well, such as the White-Light Spotlight Meditation and Waterfall Meditations.

It is focusing of your attention to receiving PE from above you that initiates this process. You may have Embracing/Conducting Heaven spontaneously during prayer and/or another spiritual experiences. Usually people hold out there hands, palms to the sky and have even been known to rock back and forth in a wave

---

[63] Most religious practices have a different perspective of doing this, although I see the nature of the process as the same.

motions as the energies of heaven flow into and threw them.

Some people have been even known to start shaking, such as the religious groups called "Shakers/Quakers". I have witnessed people in both movements and have experienced them directly as well. The waving is like being caught up in powerful waves of PE. Shaking has been associated with releasing unhealthy PE, as well as physical congestion. This is often being simulated in energy healing-empowerment treatments, massage and other treatments to help get the psychic and physical energy flowing again. In Asian and other practices, bouncing on the spot is done for these benefits, commonly known as "The Cure for a Thousand Illnesses".

Conducting/Embracing Heaven Exercise

In a meditative state, hold your hands up in front of you, palms facing up with the intention of PE flowing down upon you. Let them wash threw you, carrying away unhealthy PE and filling you with healthy PE. Let your hands go to where they naturally are drawn to go, whether this be reaching above your head, in front of your heart/fourth chakra or facing a part of your body. Trust your intuition.

Conducting Heaven can be made into Embracing Heaven by simply having the intent to embracing these energies more than channeling them into the Earth. These two exercises are usually used together in different proportions, depending on the moment. Let it happen naturally.

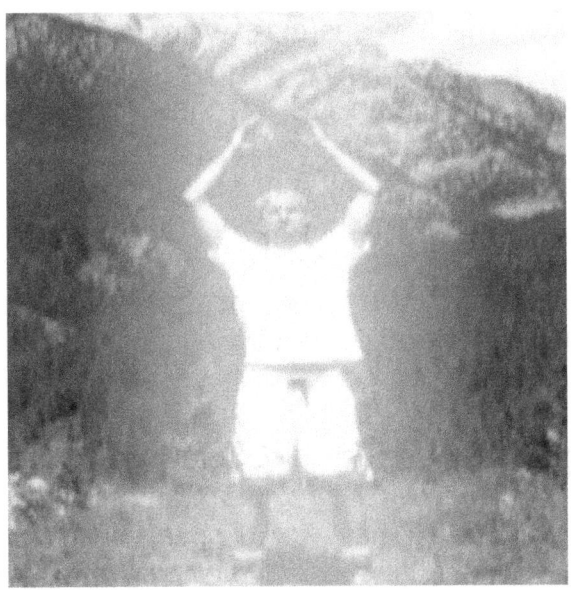

Figure 42: Shows Conducting Heaven Exercise

Embracing/Conducting Earth

Embracing Earth is also a popular technique in many qi-gong and martial practices as well; not so much in religious practices. It is usually done by focusing on connecting your tan tein through your hara line to the Earth. This is a powerful and direct way compared to connect to the Earth.

Other techniques for Embracing Earth include visualizing roots coming out of your feet tapping into the Earth. Another is using your root chakra and/or vessels to draw upon Earth energies, which I find very vitalizing. Just doing physical things can help connect you to the Earth and draw energies from it.

When connecting to the inside of Earth, the idea is to focus the healthy energies in your psychic anatomy into the Earth to resonant with Earth energies and then embrace those Earth energies into your psychic anatomy. This gives strength and stability to your healthy energies, which is really important if they are predominantly based on more spiritual parts of you. For example, lots of the healthy energies from your practice will exist predominantly on the more spiritual parts of yourself, because they originate from your soul and beyond. Naturally, they descend towards being embodied on more physical parts of you, such as the crystalline structure of your physical body (ex. DNA). By learning to resonant these energies with Earth energies, they can more powerfully influence the more physical parts of you.

People who do not practice Embracing Earth or another grounding technique usually get weak body's after many years of spiritual practice. They would spend much of their time feeling "spacey", because most of their unconscious attention is with PE far from their physical body.

It is easy to get and stay ungrounded, spiritual experiences are awesome! You must make it a priority to be grounded in the here and now with your these enlightened states still being experienced. Easier said than done in the beginning, I know. I still find myself unbalanced in this way time to time. Rest a sure, it is well worth the effort to embody these enlightened states while being grounded.

Embracing/Conducting Earth Exercise

In a meditative state, hold your hands in front of you, palms facing the Earth with the intentions of PE flowing up from the Earth into you (Embracing Earth). Let the PE from the Earth resonate with the PE in your entire being that help you live to your fullest potential. This will help them become stronger within you. Doing this to help ground yourself before, during and after the psychic energy practices is highly recommended.

Embracing Earth can be made into Conducting Earth by simply having the intent to conduct these energies into the sky. Surrounding the Earth are etheric grids that you might become aware of when doing this. Conducting Heaven can also involve these grids time to time. These two exercises (Embracing and Conducting Earth) are usually used together in different proportions, depending on the moment. It happens naturally.

Conducting Earth can be more of a workout for your psychic anatomy. If it feels better to only Embrace Earth, then please do so. Always trust how you are feeling when practicing Psychic Anatomy Yoga.

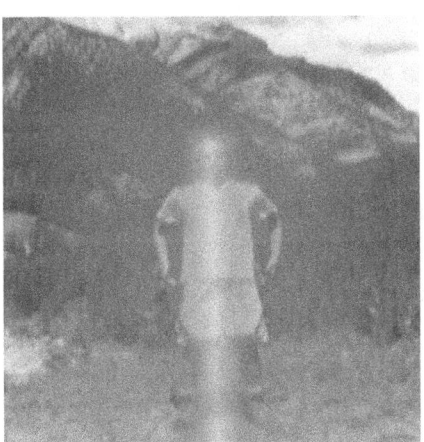 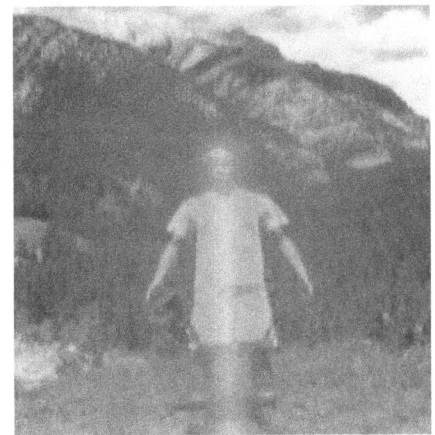

Figure 43: Shows Embracing Earth

Bridging Heaven and Earth

Bridging Heaven and Earth is a popular technique in many qi-gong and martial practices as well. Essentially it is Embracing/Conducting Heaven and Embracing/Conducting Earth at the same time. In general, it is best to do the Heaven and Earth Exercises in these ways. It will help empower the heaven energies with Earth energies and help reshape the Earth energies with heaven energies to more specifically facilitate your development.

Remember that there is more to you than your human consciousness. When it comes to psychic energy practices, your higher-self and spirit guides/angels can help more easily. Such as by reshaping psychic energy patterns as just discussed and helping you get connected to them.

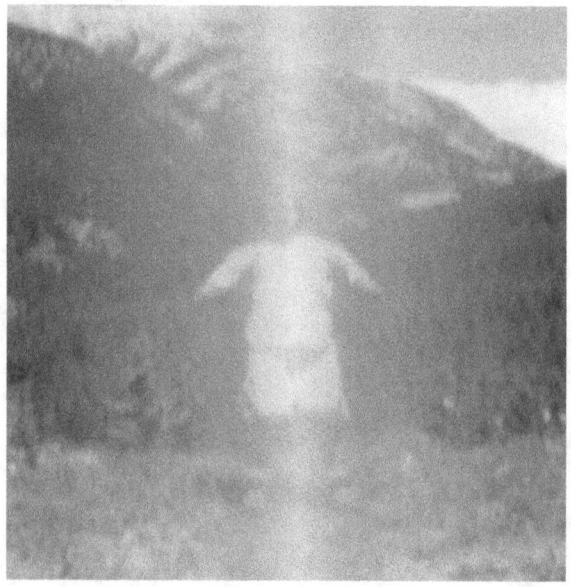

Figure 44: Shows the Bridging of Heaven and Earth

Arm Movements that Compliment Heaven and Earth Exercises

I didn't include these movements in the examples above to keep them simpler. There are two arm movement options. One is very common in qi-gong and the other in yoga. They both combine breath and movement.

Start by connecting to Earth with your hands at the bottom of your reach, palms facing the Earth or your first chakra. Focus on creating resonance with the healthy PE within and around you. On an inhalation raise your hands up, palms facing the center line of your body as you Embrace and/or Conduct Earth. When you reach the top of your reach, start to exhale with your palms now facing upwards.

Keep your hands up for as long as you like as you Embrace and/or Conduct Earth. When ready, focus on connecting to the healthy PE of heaven. On an inhalation, start to bring your hands back down, palms facing your center line as you Embrace and/or Conduct Heaven. It is common to continue Embracing and/or Conducting Earth as you bring your hands down.

When nearing the bottom of your reach, slowly turn your palms to face the Earth once again. Once in this original position, continue Embracing and/or Conducting Heaven, focusing on connecting to health Earth PE for the next cycle.

These movements are very common in qi-gong, which are essentially a form of Scanning[64]. You can also spread your arms wide, spreading the vitality of the healthy Earth and/or heaven PE into your psychic anatomy that surrounds your physical body and/or environment. These movements are common in yoga, which are essentially a form of Sweeping[65].

Final Comments

The Heaven and Earth Exercises can also be done in the background of the exercises presented in Chapters 4-7. This may sound challenging, but with a bit of practice most people pick it up.

---

[64] A General Technique.

[65] A General Technique, emphasis on spreading rather than clearing, although both can happen at the same time.

When doing Heaven and Earth Exercises with the exercises in Chapters 4-7, those parts of your psychic anatomy get more involved, which intensifies their exposure to these energies, enhancing their health and performance faster, as well as exercising them more intensely.

The Heaven and Earth Exercises are very important to Psychic Anatomy Yoga. The Heaven and Earth Exercises will likely become the climax points of your practice as intense streams of PE expand your psychic anatomy and consciousness. Remember to develop a good foundation in your psychic anatomy before aiming to have these experiences. Such power without a good foundation can be an unpleasant experience if you get overwhelmed.

Using asanas to help ground yourself and integrate with these energies after such experiences works very well. This is why combining Psychic Anatomy Exercises[66] with yoga asanas is such an incredible combination!

When you feel you have done enough of the Heaven and Earth Exercises, it is best to finish with your palms facing the Earth to help ground, balance and harmonize yourself. Remember that all it takes is the intention to be grounded, balanced and harmonized to initiate the process.

It is best to gain some experience with these exercises in routines involving the exercises in Chapters 4-7, and on their own before moving on to the next chapter. If you would like to combine them with your yoga asana practice, please do so when you are standing (ex. between heat series/sun salutations). There are other opportunities to use these exercises as well, which I will discuss in Section ?. For now keep it simple and develop a good foundation.

---

[66] *The Psychic Anatomy Exercises* teaches larger set of psychic energy exercises.

CHAPTER 11
SOME FINAL EXERCISES

General Alignment

Once you do get the hang of working with your psychic anatomy as discussed in Chapters 4-7, you can start to balance and harmonize all of them together. The idea is to hold more and more of your psychic anatomy in your awareness at once as you focus healthy PE upon it and intend/visualize it being balanced and harmonized.

This is an advanced exercise. You are not expected to start using it right away. It could take several months before you are ready and that is perfectly fine. It is like driving a car, in time it gets much easier. Start small and progress. In time you will be able to hold your entire psychic anatomy in alignment. When the health and performance of your psychic anatomy is well developed, this can be a very powerful and quick technique to align your psychic anatomy and charge it with healthy PE.

I recommend doing a General Alignment every morning and every night. Doing it during the day can help you stay focused on your priorities and achieve them well. Once you get good at it, it can take less than a minute and make a significant difference to how you feel.

Once you can do this exercise and maintain it, you can try maintaining it during other activities, such as your Psychic Anatomy Yoga practice. Might sound out of reach, but it is gets fairly easy once you get the hang of it. It helps to stay very relaxed and make it your priority over challenging asanas.

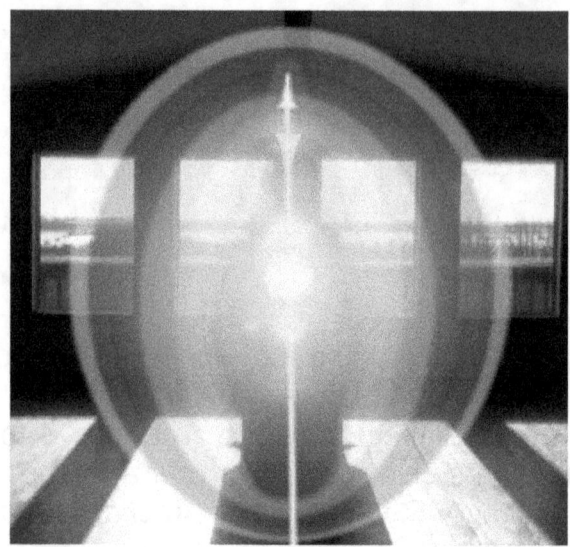

Figure 45: Shows a General Alignment with all parts of psychic anatomy, excluding the meridians and internal aura.

Turning Inwards

Religious and mystic teachers have also taught us to look inward to find God. The ancient Hindis believed that our soul is the incarnation of an over-soul, and this over-soul is the incarnation of another over-soul (over-soul 2). This pattern repeats itself all the way back to God/Atma[67]. By turning inwards into your core star and soul gates, you can develop this connection more easily.

Turning outwards can help you do this as well, but remember that the goal is to establish your connection to God, not to reference another being that is better connected. These being's can be very helpful, but only to help you develop your own connections.

---

[67]   The omnipresence/soul of all souls.

Turning Inwards can lead you towards very powerful experiences, but only when you are ready for them. If you try and are not ready, your experiences will not likely be as rewarding. I recommend everything I teach as preparation for empowering and furthering this connection.

Your soul gate can send you PE from your soul and your higher soul gates (ex. soul gate 2, soul gate 3, etc) can send you PE from your over souls. It takes time to develop the ability to work with your soul gates. Be patient in this process as a good foundation makes for better results and faster growth.

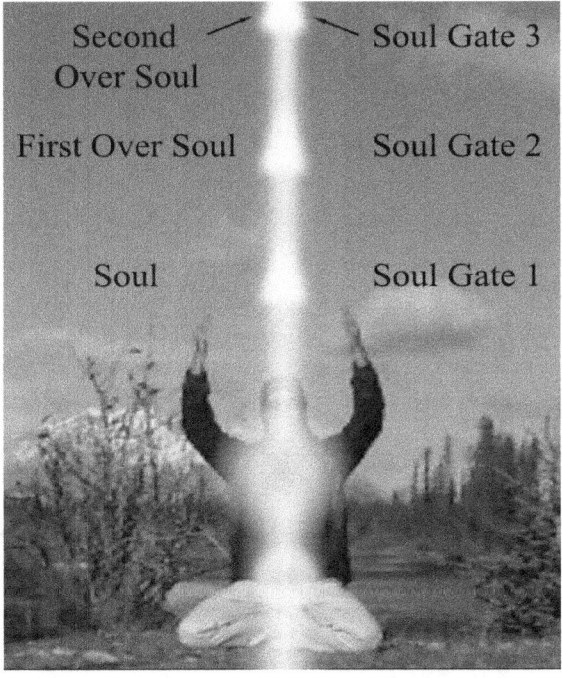

Figure 46: Shows the Hara with Soul Gates 2 and 3 included. There are higher Soul Gates as well.

Ultimately this exercise results in your soul gate(s) sending PE towards your physical body to help prepare your psychic anatomy and physical body to embody PE of a more enlightened nature. This involves the crystalline structures in your body changing to hold resonance with these energies, such as your DNA[68].

Your soul gates can also send PE directly into your core star. This is usually a process of more of your soul incarnating, which means you are doing well. Your psychic anatomy and physical body need to be in a good state of health and performance to handle large quantities of soul energy. Again, it has to do with resonance as discussed at the end of the last paragraph.

I have experienced this as my core star expanding and becoming more dense. There have been times when after this expansion, part of it collapsed and became much brighter as a transparent glow expanded to create an orb of light around my aura.

Start with an Experiential Meditation, focus on being connected to your soul gate(s), use your hands to help empower these centers and then moving into Heaven and Earth Exercises or Ascending/Descending (discussed below). Doing a General Alignment before this exercise is recommended. Doing a General Alignment with this exercise is also recommended.

Ascending/Descending

Ascending/Descending are powerful concepts that are the climax of psychic energy exercises in Psychic Anatomy Yoga. They are also the most advanced, relaying on you being able to

---

[68] I discuss this in a few books, particularly in *The Interface Between Psychic Energies and the Physical Body*, where I go into lots of scientific detail.

do a General Alignment and work with all parts of your psychic anatomy. The concept is to Ascend more physically based PE (ex. Earth energies) towards your soul gates and core star. This empowers your psychic anatomy one part at a time, starting with its most physically based parts towards its most spiritually based parts (ex. meridians, to first chakra and auric body, towards seventh chakra and auric body, to the hara line's connection to Earth, towards soul gates, to core star). This is best done while holding a General Alignment, although in is not necessary.

Ascending more physically based PE helps strengthen your psychic anatomy, making it easier to handle more power and flow from more spiritually based PE. When restrictions are met on the path of Ascending, they can be addressed in the moment or passed over and returned to later.

Descending is the same concept, but uses more spiritually based PE and in reverse (ex. core star to soul gates, towards hara line's connection to the Earth, to seventh chakra and auric body, towards first chakra and auric body to meridians). When restrictions are met on the path of Descending PE, they can be addressed in the moment or passed over and returned to later as well.

Descending is a very powerful concept, because it empowers a natural process. Your soul, over souls and spirit guides[69] send you PE from more spiritual aspects of creation to help you evolve. By empowering this process, it makes it easier for the energies they send to make it to their destinations. The more physically based these targets are, the harder it is for them to be reached well. The better state of health and performance your psychic anatomy is in, the easier it is for them to reach these targets. Descending facilitates this process greatly as well!

---

[69] There maybe other sources as well.

The exercises in Chapters 4-7 help clear and expand the path, General Alignment helps straighten it and Descending helps empower it. Descending, as well as Ascending, can be done with the Heaven and Earth Exercises for more power. By focusing on Heaven and/or Earth energies tuning to those that you are naturally working with before Ascending/Descending, the process can be more effective[70].

The geometry of your physical anatomy, from entire organs to molecules, play a role in how well you embody/resonant with certain vibrations of PE. DNA is the best example and the most important. Descending PE all the way to it, visualizing it integrating with them will help empower the process, resulting in change to gene expression and your genetic code.

Learning to work with your Internal Aura and physical anatomy greatly helps to reach these deeper parts of you, such as your DNA and other biocrystals. Your internal aura is the aura under your skin, your meridians actually help support it. Descending PE into your internal aura helps empower it with the Descending PE[71]. I discuss working with your internal aura and physical body in more depth in Level 5 within *The Psychic Anatomy Exercises*. I highly recommend it!

As your body evolves to resonant with the PE you are growing into, general health and performance can/will improve, but even more importantly, you are helping your body to embody more of your soul, which is a big part of enlightenment. The more of your soul you embody, the more you become aware of and powerful with PE. This is a major part of your/our evolution and the meaning of life.

Wow is an understatement! ;)

---

[70] I discusses periodically in *The Psychic Anatomy Exercises*.

[71] I discuss the internal aura in more depth within *The Psychic Energy Reality, The Interface between Psychic Energies and the Physical Body* and with exercises in *The Psychic Anatomy Exercises*.

This is the most advanced technique, be patient with developing your foundation before exploring it. When you start to explore it, be mindful of using it until it happens spontaneously. Your intuition should be well developed by the time this happens, so you will not need to question it. Once it happens spontaneously a few time, you will be ready top use it more willingly.

Cycling

Cycling is a technique I have discussed before. Its the repeating of exercises or sequences of exercises. For example, Ascending then Descending, then Ascending again.

The benefits of this technique come from changes that occur as you progress with an exercise or sequence of exercises. When changes occur, parts of you that have already been addressed may be able to change more easily. By Cycling/repeating exercises (sometimes in reverse order {ex. Chakra Exercise 1-7 then Chakra Exercise 7-1}), these parts get addressed a second, third or fourth time. How many times you Cycle is up to you.

In general, it is best to keep Cycling until a smooth sequence is completed, meaning no areas that need extra attention are found. In the beginning this may not be possible, but as you progress, most routines will follow this pattern.

General Routine

This is the general routine I recommend. Psychic Anatomy Yoga can incorporate breaks using asanas, which needs to be mindfully timed. I'll give an example of this in the next subsection.

Start by doing a General Alignment with Scanning and Intuitive

Movements to facilitate the General Alignment. When you feel aligned, Conduct/Embrace Earth and then include Conducting/Embracing Heaven. Continue with the Heaven and Earth Exercises as you see fit. When ready, start Ascending from the first region of your aura towards your core star. This is intended to help prepare you for Descending. If you practice a lot, you may be able to combine Ascending with your General Alignment.

Once you are done with your core star, raise your hands above your head to face your soul gate(s) and do Pulsate Breathing to help empower them. Scanning/Sweeping down your hara line/chakra column can help bring the PE they radiate into the parts of your psychic anatomy below. When ready, Descend with the intent of facilitating the integration of the PE coming from your soul gate(s) and core star.

While doing this, some parts will receive more attention than others and some will not receive any attention at all. In the beginning, give every part of your psychic anatomy some attention. How far you Descend is up to you. Sometimes it will only be to the first region of your aura and other time it will be all the way into your internal aura, cells and DNA. You will know how far to go intuitively.

When you have finished Descending, start another Cycle beginning at your core star or Ascending back towards it. Ascending is always a safe and wise choice, but sometimes, especially as you develop, it will not be necessary.

In general, as you continue to Cycle, less and less parts of your psychic anatomy will need extra attention. You will likely spend more time sweeping the PE down and threw your psychic anatomy to the parts that need it, using General Techniques to facilitate the natural processes. These parts will likely be more physically based as they are denser forms of energy, which makes them harder to change/upgrade.

In this process, your fourth charka will play a more dominant role by creating and sustaining a connection/relationship with the PE you are Descending (recall the fourth chakra works with the PE of relationships). Your seventh and first chakras will also get more involved as the descending PE enter your seventh chakras directly and go directly to your first charka/region to help create resonance with more physically based PE. This will more powerfully influence your vessels, meridians and internal aura (internal aura includes physical body), which is where the change needs to happen to fully embody higher state of consciousness. Your body is a crystalline antenna for PE[72].

It is common for the tan tien to be more involved as well, particularly near the end, because it can help remove unwanted and establish wanted psychic energy memories[73]. Remember to be mindful when Ascending, because the changes could be sensitive to the denser Earth PE. This means it may take longer to Ascend the Earth PE that help empower these changes. As the integration process completes itself, you will naturally start to Ascend PE more intensely, building strength.

As you advance, try giving more attention to doing the Heaven and Earth Exercises as you follow the General Routine. This will help empower the Ascending/Descending processes. Also try giving more attention to the presence of the PE of virtues (Rays). You may become aware of specific virtues that you are integrating with. This awareness will help empower them more directly, because awareness is a way of focusing your attention[74].

---

[72] Discussed in scientific detail within *The Interface Between Psychic Energies and the Physical Body;* details on this interface in regards to the brain.

[73] Recall tan tien helps anchor PE into the aura.

[74] The power of being a witness.

General Routine with Asanas

When practicing a General Routine, you can include asanas in between segments of the routine. This can be a very beneficial thing to do, because it will help ground you, as well as make it easier for PE to flow threw your physical body. PE need to flow threw your physical body to influence the internal aura, as well as to help release unhealthy PE.

In general, doing at least one complete system of your psychic anatomy (ex. hara system) between sets of asanas is recommended. I encourage you to do more as well. Make the psychic energy exercises of Part 1 your priority and use asanas to compliment them.

Final Comments

When practicing these and other exercises involving PE, remember to stay in a meditation state afterward to focus on balancing and harmonizing your mind, body and spirit (physical body and psychic anatomy). During this time, visions, insights and spontaneous PE experiences can happen. These spontaneous PE experiences usually come from natural processes in your psychic anatomy, as well as your soul and/or spirit guides[75] working with you.

It is very rare to have negative spirits around you, but some people do. If it feels like there are unhealthy PE trying to interact with you, turn your attention inwards as you amplify your positive energy. The brighter you shine the better. It will drown out the influences around you, attract resonant PE, as well as help transmute/neutralize unhealthy PE.

---

[75] Spirit guides are usually advanced souls that didn't incarnate and have decided to help you with your incarnation. Some of them are soul family.

Sometimes these feelings come from within, which is sourced by an inner issue(s) you are not in touch with. These exercises will help surface them as a natural consequence of healthier PE causing unhealthy ones to be detoxified. You can basically do the same thing to help purify yourself of them. Being aligned to the higher aspects of your consciousness (ex. soul and over-souls), especially the soul of all souls (aka. Omnipresent state/God) is a very powerful alignment!.

Sometimes these issues are dissolved without really experiencing them and other times they are. The more you practice the faster they will be detoxed and the better you will get at detoxifying them.

Sometimes they will be difficult to detox. In these situations I recommend *Inner and Outer Success* for a review of the best of conventional self-help techniques and many involving PE. I also recommend working with other people, such as Energy Psychologist and/or Energy Healing/Empowerment practitioners. A little/lot of support can go a long way!

Doing Psychic Anatomy Yoga in groups can help as well, because these groups increase the power, harmony and diversity of PE to work with, which is sometimes enough to detox inner issues more easily. More on practicing with groups in Appendix A.

It is common for intuition to guide you (Intuitive Movements) as you practice. Please trust it! You are your greatest teacher in Psychic Anatomy Yoga. I am only here to help you develop your foundation. It is you who will lead your way to greatness!

Remember to finish your practice feeling grounded. Use the techniques already presented to help connect to and empower yourself with Earth PE. You have incarnated on Earth for a reason. Build your relationship with the healthier aspects of being here to help empower yourself for your life's purpose.

CHAPTER 12
FINAL COMMENTS ON PART 1

There has been enough information presented to keep you developing the health and performance of your psychic anatomy for years. As you get better at doing the exercises presented, you'll become more aware of details and be able to empower yourself more specifically and generally.

To get faster results and more powerful experiences, practice these exercises in a group. Groups work together to draw in a greater diversity of PE, which also tend to be more powerful and harmonized as well. Group experiences can be truly amazing! Especially when a few experienced people are present.

As you develop your psychic anatomy's health and performance on your own and/or with a group, you'll still need to make time to maintain your physical health. It is as easy as having healthy eating and sleeping routines, as well as getting your heart rate up for at least 10 minutes a day. See *A Formula for Evolution/God's Journey* and *Becoming Super Human* for details on these topics.

Psychic Anatomy Yoga can be your heart rate exercise, but most people's heart rate actually decrease. Either way, getting your heart rate up after practicing asanas is a good idea, because it helps flush out the toxins that get released as a consequence of stretching. It also helps deliver nutrients to different parts of the body. It is best to involve your arms and legs when getting your heart rate up, such as with a cross trainer or walking with your arms pumping, because it helps with circulation. You will also need sufficient water in your body for this to work optimally.

If you are interested in learning more or having difficulties understanding the psychic energy exercises and/or psychic anatomy in this book, please see my book *The Psychic Anatomy Exercises* for a more detailed descriptions of psychic anatomy and some additional exercises.

Part 2 will discuss some unique insights on yoga asanas and how psychic energy techniques can be included with them.

PART 2

INCORPORATING ASANAS

CHAPTER 13
INTRODUCTION

This section describes the combination of the psychic energy exercises from Part 1 with yoga asanas, giving you Psychic Anatomy Yoga.

I commented in the beginning of this book that the roots of yoga were more focused on PE than modern day teachings are. Kundalini and Tantra yoga practices still maintain some of these teachings, but I my opinion, most of it has been lost. Psychic Anatomy Yoga revives the focus of PE with psychic energy exercises based upon many traditional and scientific perspectives from around the world[76].

I'll make some comments on the techniques discussed in Part 1 before moving onto the asanas. General Alignments can be done very quickly once you get the hang of them, which will help prepare your psychic anatomy to get the most out of your practice. Always do a General Alignment before you start your practice. It can also be beneficial to do at the end of your practice while focusing on integrating, balancing and harmonizing with the changes that have occurred.

The Heaven and Earth Exercises are good to do near the beginning of your practice to help expand, clear and empower your psychic anatomy, preparing to do psychic energy exercises more effectively. Doing Heaven and Earth exercises periodically during your practice can help reinforce these benefits, as well as enhance other exercises when they are combined with them. For example, doing an Heaven and Earth Exercises while Ascending or Descending.

---

[76] See *The Psychic Energy Reality* for a review of this information.

Standing and sitting are excellent opportunities for spending longer periods of time doing the psychic energy exercises of Part 1. Some asanas, such as Tree, Standing Lunge, Warrior 1, Warrior 2 and others, are good opportunities for doing them for shorter periods of time. I'll discuss these asanas in the chapters that follow.

It is up to you to decide how many psychic energy exercises to include in your Psychic Anatomy Yoga practice. At first, start with a few, following the order they are given in this book and progress as you see fit. Remember that it takes time to develop a good foundation, and good foundations are important to your optimal development.

Doing too many psychic energy exercises or doing them too powerfully[77], can leave you feeling overwhelmed, especially if you forcing yourself to do them when you are tired or not experienced with them. It can also happen if you practice often and do not give enough attention to balancing, harmonizing and grounding yourself. Always make balancing, harmonizing and being grounded your first priorities.

Build a good foundation with the psychic energy exercises in Chapters 4-7 and General Alignments before using Ascending/Descending and the Heaven and Earth Exercises powerfully. This will give you the best results (quality before quantity). You can still do these exercises as you develop your foundation. They actually play an important role in developing it. You just need to be mindful of how powerfully and often you do them. In the beginning, such power does not commonly exist, but as you develop your skills with Psychic Anatomy Yoga, your power will increase.

Psychic Anatomy Yoga techniques can take you out of your body, weakening it temporarily until you ground yourself and

---

[77] PE are controlled by attention. Focus your attention intensely and the associated PE will get more intense.

the enlightened PE you have cultivated. This is one of the reasons why Psychic Anatomy Yoga is such a great practice. As you connect to higher states of consciousness and associated PE, you are immediately grounding yourself and associated PE using asanas.

The asanas will not always be enough. Getting your heart rate up after practice for ten minutes will help ground you even more, as well as help flush fresh blood threw your muscles and body in general, carrying away waste materials and supplying nutrients[78]. Walking in nature and/or working with vegetation (ex. gardening) are other options to help ground you as well as provide other benefits associated with vegetation[79].

The next chapter discusses some physical aspects of an asana practice that I find important. I will discuss some of these topics and others in the chapters that follow as well. This book is not intended to teach you how to do asanas. To learn about about doing asanas, I recommend "Kirtpula Yoga" by Faulds and senior teachers at the Kirtpula Yoga Institute and looking online for credible resources[80].

---

[78] Stretching and healthy PE cause toxins to be detoxed.
[79] Humans have a symbiotic relationship with vegetation in physical and psychic energy ways.
[80] Most will be fine, but Yoga Institutions are usually better.

CHAPTER 14
ON THE PHYSICAL TOPICS OF ASANAS

Yoga asanas are know for combining breath and movement in a mindful-meditative state of being. There are some other important teachings that I will review below that you may or may not already be aware of. I do not comment on getting in and out of asanas, proper posture in them or breathing in regards to asanas much. There are many good books that do this. I recommend "Kirtpula Yoga" by Faulds and senior teachers at the Kirtpula Yoga Institute and looking online for credible resources[81].

Cardiovascular Exercise

Doing at least 5-10 minutes of cardiovascular exercise before practice helps to oxygenate your muscles, which will help you be stronger in your practice and get deeper into asanas. Doing at least 5-10 minutes afterward will help flush your muscles and body of toxins released during your practice, as well as help deliver nutrients. It is more important to do cardiovascular exercise after class for these reasons.

Be mindful after practice, because your muscles and body could be overly fatigued, causing cardiovascular exercise to do more harm than good. In these situations, I recommend rejuvenating for a while with water, electrolytes, sugar and free amino acids[82]. Fruit is a great choice, because it contains water, sugar and other nutrients that will energize and help detoxify the body. Free amino acids, especially branch-chained, glutamate

---

[81] Most will be fine, but Yoga Institutions are usually better.

[82] Free amino acids mean they are not a part of a protein, which allows them to be absorbed by the body almost immediately.

and beta-alanine amino acids will help aid in vitality and recovery[83].

If your class was very intense, doing 5-10 minute sessions periodically during the day (maybe the next day as well) is recommended to keep flushing your muscles and organs. Remember, this doesn't need to be a workout, just enough to get your heart pumping for 5-10 minutes.

Some will argue that a yoga practice should get your heart rate up. I agree that this is true in some situations, but not all. Yoga can be a very meditative experience, which will actually lower your heart rate. When it comes to Psychic Anatomy Yoga this is even more likely to happen. This is not to imply your body doesn't get worked hard. In deeper meditative states, especially when PE are involved, the body can work very hard and not experience strain[84].

> Sometimes when you are tired, cardiovascular exercise is just what you need to free the stagnant energy that is making you feel tired.

Neck and Upper-Mid Back

Some yoga practices need more neck and upper back attention. Your neck is a pivotal point in your posture. If it is tight, postural misalignment can create tension elsewhere in the body. It is as easy as bringing one ear to a shoulder with some variations as you pull your opposite shoulder down. Doing this three times a day, gently at first, until you learn your neck's

---

[83] Discussed in *Becoming Super Human* with other topics of advanced nutrition.
[84] Another example of this is discussed in Hunt, 1989, *Infinite Mind,* p. 12.

limits, will give you awesome results, especially if energy healing, massage and/or hot-cold flushes are incorporated as well. Be mindful, because you can over-stretch your neck easily with the power of your back pulling your shoulder down.

As your neck starts to release, it will become easier to do asanas that target your upper and mid back. These areas are where most people store PE associated with stress, causing muscles and tendon tension there. By stretching them with asanas (ex. Thread the Needle variations discussed in Chapter 16), you can expect great releases over time in these areas, which can be an incredible feeling!

It is possible to experience temporary discomfort as particular muscles release and others stay tight. Be persistent and mindful, because this is not the time to take a long break. You need to continue to practice to help maintain the release in these muscles and encourage the release in the others. This is a great time to incorporate Energy Healing, massage and/or hot-cold flushes to facilitate the process.

Hands, Wrists and Forearms

Hands, wrists and forearms are used every day. If you press upon your forearms, you'll likely find numerous muscles that feel tight and maybe even knotted. By helping these parts get healthier with self massage, acupressure and stretching, you'll find more comfort and capability when using them for physical and psychic energy purposes. It will also help protect you from future problems in these areas, such as arthritis.

Hand stretches can be done by stretching the fingers back one at a time and pulling them forward. Afterward, expanding and clenching your hand periodically and/or rubbing your stretched fingers, hand and forearm, you'll help flush fresh blood threw them. This is an important concept, because these areas tend to have limited blood circulation.

There are lots of opportunities for wrist stretches in an asana routine. You can stretch the inside of them by pressing your hands down while in prayer. You can move your hands towards and away from your body to target them from different angles as well. The outside of can be done in a similar way.

Your forearms get stretched by wrist stretches to a degree. I find that by resisting the wrist stretches engages more of my forearm muscles. Be mindful not to resist too greatly so you avoid possible strains.

Feet, Ankles, Calves and Shins

Feet, ankles, calves and shins are also very important when it comes to balance and being grounded. These parts of you can be treated the same way as your hands, wrists and forearms.

Your feet can have their toes stretched the same way you do your fingers. Remember to rub them afterward as well. Feet are very special when it comes to being rubbed and reflexology. Taking good care of your could make a significant difference to the health and performance of your entire body.

Your feet are also pivotal points in your posture; similar to your neck. If tension inhibits proper posture at your base, other parts of the body can get tight as they compensate.

Your ankles will need extra attention, because they are not stretched well when working on your feet. Using a foam block under your knees while leaning back can help stretch the front of your ankles and shins. The back of your ankles and calves can be done in Down Dog variations. For example, bending your knees a bit to target your calves more and changing the angle of your feet to target the sides of your calves. Concepts of variations discussed below.

Resisting/Engaging

Resisting, also know as engaging, helps intensify the stretch as well as build strength. Sometimes resisting is needed to help target tight muscles that are not easily targeted by asanas alone. Try going into Child's Pose and pulling your spine out of your hips as much as you can. Now start to resist with torso slowly (flex/engage it). You will notice how it pulls your spine out of your hips even more.

You can also slowly resist with your hips and legs, which I find helps create a more balanced distribution of the tension, as well as intensifies it. This approach might help improve posture as well, because your muscles are holding you in place, rather than the pressure on your joints. For example, when resisting in Down Dog, you can feel how the distribution of tension threw your hips changes.

When exploring resisting/engaging, be mindful not to strain yourself. There are many small muscles I your body that could take the bulk of the tension from resisting/engaging.

Centering Your Spine

The title of this concept can be applied in two ways. There is a conventional concept of being balanced on left and right sides of your body and there is the concept of centering your spine with the center of your body, essentially pulling it inwards, towards your chakra column and hara line. Opening your hips helps a lot for doing this.

It takes a lot of practice for the body to learn to reposition the spine more inwardly. It has many benefits to strength, posture and psychic anatomy. Back bends take on a whole new experience when being mindful of this.

Static and Dynamic Variations

Static and dynamic variations, such as twists and rotations of your limbs and/or torso to get a more comprehensive stretch and strengthening are almost necessary to get a comprehensive workout from asanas. For example, in Down Dog[85] or Forward Fold[86], you can rotate the direction of your feet, lean into one of your legs, lift one foot at a time and more to target different angles of your body.

Often reaching and resisting will be helpful for getting the most out of these variations. In static variations, you can simply engage muscles to create enough tension to target tight muscles effectively. This is especially true for the smaller muscles that are not easy to notice until exploring variations. Do this carefully to avoid strain.

Other examples are given below, but the options are really endless. It takes your initiative to mindfulness find what works best for you.

Twisting and leaning are the most common static variations, which are great for stretching and strengthening core muscles, while squeezing the organs and muscles. They are also easy to incorporate into almost any asana.

Less common is the twisting of arms and wrists. For example, twisting one extended arm in one direction and the other in the opposite can be done slowly for stretching and strengthening, or more quickly for toning and awakening the shoulders (imagine your arm(s) as being wrung like a wet towel). You can even include your shoulders and spine into the variation. When

---

[85] Discussed in Chapter 19.
[86] Discussed in Chapter 18.

doing this, reaching out of your shoulders and/or resisting will make these movements more intense. Remember to be mindful of your limits when exploring these options. This example can be used as a dynamic variation as well; discussed below.

Correct posture for an asana is over-emphasized in some teachings. Sometimes you need to bend a knee or arch your back to target important areas. When moving into/finding these variations, move slowly for two reasons. First of all, it is safer. Secondly, it will help you find the areas that need the most attention.

You'll sometimes find areas that are close together and not relaxed/lengthened the same, causing a noticeable difference when passing over them. Target the tighter area mindfully and try to bring them into the same state of relaxation/length. Sometimes you'll not be able to move through these areas fully and you'll need to decrease the stretch and pass over them, returning to them later from a different angle or maybe relaxing another area will help it to relax[87].

These variations can be very empowering and intense in regards to PE. PE can be stored in these areas as a result of the mind-body-spirit connection. When they are targeted, great healing can be triggered. It is likely you've experienced such healing in standard asanas when your body first started opening up in a certain way. Many you have experienced this with a form of physical therapy. When it happens, keep drawing in healthy PE to help the release occur and for general support. It can feel very good to find and work with these areas. Doing so can reduce your need for chiropractic and other physical therapies.

When coming out of such an area, there can be a lot of lactic acid released, which needs to be flushed out to reduce stiffness and discomfort later on. Increased heart rate, energy healing,

---

[87] This is a physical example of the concept of Cycling discussed in Chapter 11.

massage and hot-cold have already been discussed. I discuss a few other options below.

As you target the areas found when exploring variations, dynamic variations can be used at a lower intensity of stretch to help the area(s) realign. Creating circles with your neck, shoulders, elbow, wrists, hips, knees and ankles are all great to help muscles and tendons reposition after a release. These movements also help circulate blood, which can be very important for areas with limited blood supply.

I issue caution with dynamic and static variations, because some postures can create tension on joints and other body parts that are unhealthy. You need to be mindful of what you are doing and receptive to criticism. Remember that it is easier to see other people from a distance, even when surrounded by mirrors, which is where your criticism will be coming from.

Bouncing, Tapping and Shaking

Bouncing, tapping and shaking can help the body release and realign similar to dynamic variations, but without stretching. They can also do more. These techniques are very common in Asian practices for freeing stagnant qi/chi (aka. PE) from within the body and resorting health and vitality. Some people know bouncing on the spot as "The Cure for a Thousand Illnesses". The basic idea is that the physical vibrations help break up stagnation in the physical body and psychic anatomy.

The best way to use them is with your breath being in harmony with them. For example, let your breath carry the rhythm of your bouncing, tapping and/or shaking. Sometimes you'll need to decrease the intensity of your bouncing, tapping and/or shaking as releases occur with your breath. This is OK.

I find bouncing, tapping and shaking great for helping parts of my body release that need extra help. It can be as simple as bouncing on the balls of your feet, always staying in contact with the ground to minimize impact. Jarring impact is not always helpful and sometime unhealthy.

As you bounce, you can tap over organs, muscles, joints, meridians and meridian points with an open palm, your finger tips, both hands or one hand as you focus on using healthy PE as well. The healthy PE can be specific, such as healthy liver, happy liver, I love my liver, etc. You can also shake your body as you do this. Trust your intuition on how best to use these techniques.

Breathing

Breathing is so important! *The Miracle of Breath* states that the healthiest breathing has no pause between inhalation and exhalation with equal time spent on both. Yoga calls this Circular Breathing. Shallow circular breathing is relaxing. Deeper circular breathing is empowering and can stimulate releases in targeted areas as large amounts of prana (aka. PE) is brought in and out of the body by the lungs.

Sometimes shallow breathing can get you into a place of relaxation that facilitates a release as well. A release from this approach is usually noticed as a deep inhalation, followed by a faster deep exhalation. Allow yourself to feel comfortable in your yoga classes to let these deep exhalations out. Giving sound to such exhalations can help as well, which may or may not be appropriate in your class.

Deep exhalations can also be the release of anxiety in the moment. If so, you may be breathing predominately with your chest, your abdomen coming inwards on the inhalation. If so, focus on having your abdomen expand with your chest. This will lower anxiety, increase relaxation and decrease the amount of deep exhalations you are making.

In some asanas, it is difficult to breathe healthily. Try to though, because the stretching and strengthening of your diaphragm and rib cage will be worth it. Mind your limits though. Ribs can be sensitive to strain.

A Bandha Exercise

There are three main bandhas in yoga. The first is the pelvic floor, which is very popular. Next is the abdominal muscles, which help support the lower and mid back. The third is the neck, which has your chin pulled towards your chest as you tense the area. These bandhas are believed to concentrated PE in the areas of tension. This definitely seems to be the case. By contracting and releasing these bandhas in sequence with your breath, you can pulse the PE and blood flow threw the associated areas.

You can create bandhas anywhere in your body, from your forearms to an entire leg. It can help nourish a strained or depleted part of your body by breathing in with the area. Inhaling when contracted and exhaling when relaxed. You can include PE as well. Experiment with this concept. It will help you learn body-awareness, breath control, PE awareness[88] and the ability to breath prana (aka. PE). I discuss this in a bit more depth below.

Flushing With Fresh Blood

Flushing the entire body with cardiovascular exercise was discussed above. Flushing specific areas during your practice can also be done with massage and/or moving targeted areas.

---

[88] Also known as Extrasensory Perception or Clairvoyance.

For example, moving in and out of a postures slowly, flexing while entering and leaving them helps squeeze blood out, while relaxing when in and out of them helps let blood back in. Essentially the bandha concept discussed above.

Combining breath and movement, while increasing breath rate and depth (often happens naturally) helps increase heart rate and circulation. You can learn to do this very well as you get more in touch with your body and intuition/the moment. Combining this approach with the one in the last paragraph works very well.

Even just focusing on the flushing to happen will attract the associated PE that helps make it happen (manifest it). It will also bring complimentary PE as well, helping the flushing to occur in other ways (ex. flushing of unhealthy PE). Learning to use PE is a very powerful tool.

Final Comments

The following chapters are categorized as linking asanas, meaning those that are commonly used to take you in and out of other asanas. This is intended to make it easier to look them up and consider options to include in your practice.

The figures below make use of special effects to show PE and psychic anatomy during the asanas. Red light represents Earth PE and white light represent Heaven PE.

Most figures come from *Psychic Anatomy Yoga Vol 1* or *Psychic Anatomy Exercise Vol 2*. The DVDs are great for learning some things about this practice. Each chapter contains voice-over to explain what is being shown and related information.

CHAPTER 15
FROM SEATED PART 1

Often a yoga asana class will start and end in a seated posture. Such postures can sitting on your knees or sitting with crossed legs. In general, these postures result in poor circulation threw the legs (sitting on knees) or poor posture (sitting cross legged). Using a wooden or foam block can help take pressure off your legs when kneeling or be used to raise your hips above your knees when sitting with crossed legs, improving circulation and posture. Another option is using Kneeling Stool. (In Appendix H there is a simple design for making one that can also be used as a support block.)

It is very important to get in the habit of having these tools for helping you maintain a healthy posture when sitting. Many of the psychic energy exercises are best done while sitting with a straight spine. Discomfort and needing to move because of discomfort make it difficult to enter and stay in the deep states of meditation associated with these exercises. These tools can help greatly avoid these obstacles.

Even with the tools mentioned above, sitting for an hour or more can be uncomfortable. I don't recommend you force yourself out of ritual to sit for this long, but sometimes it will feel appropriate. In these moments I recommend staying with the stillness. There are many advantages to meditating for long periods of time.

If you do find yourself in a "meditation marathon", I recommended you incorporate some simple and easy movements to keep your body comfortable. Examples are Seated Forward Fold, Seated Twist, Seated Leans and there are

156

many others in *Tibetan Relaxation* by Tarthang Tulku[89].

Other seated postures that usually come in near the end of a yoga class are discussed in Chapter 23 (From Seated Part 2).

In general, it is best to leave a seated posture on to your Hands and Knees. From here there are many gentle body awakening asanas you can do.

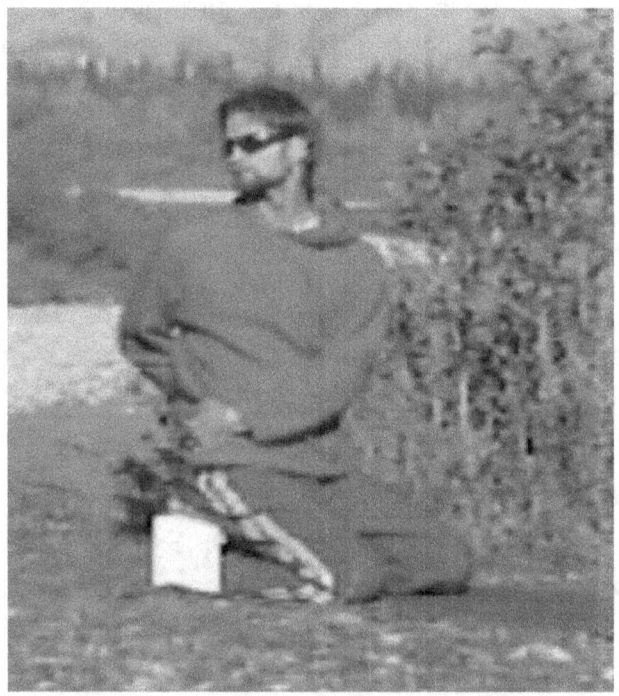

Figure 47: An example of Twist from seated.

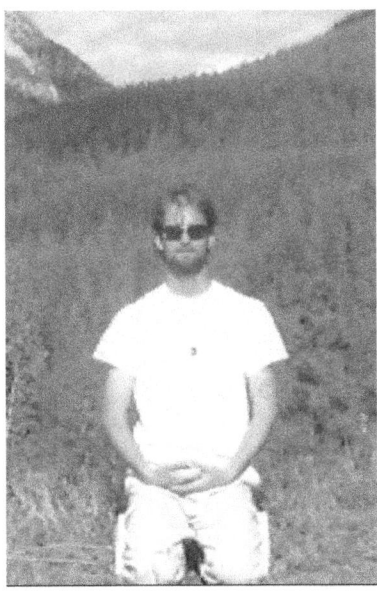 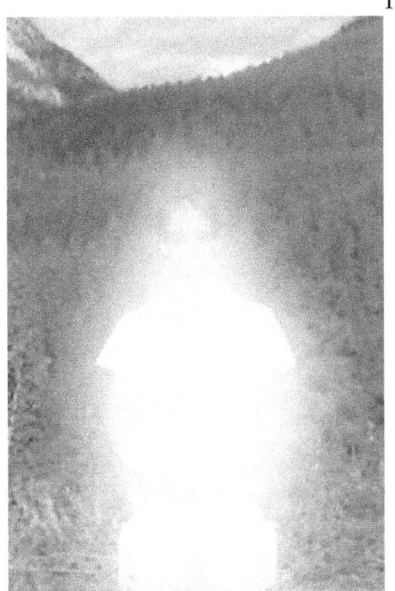

Figure 48: Shows kneeling on a kneeling stool. The right side shows the focusing of attention on charging up with healthy PE.

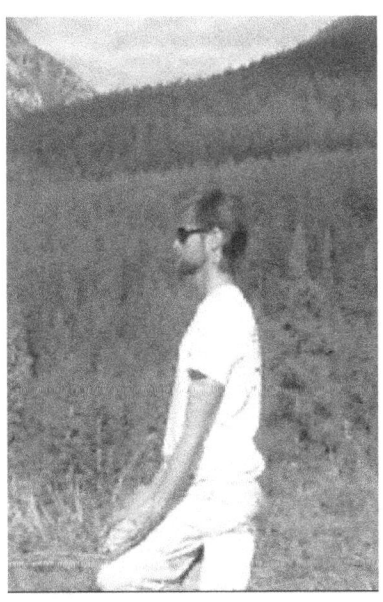 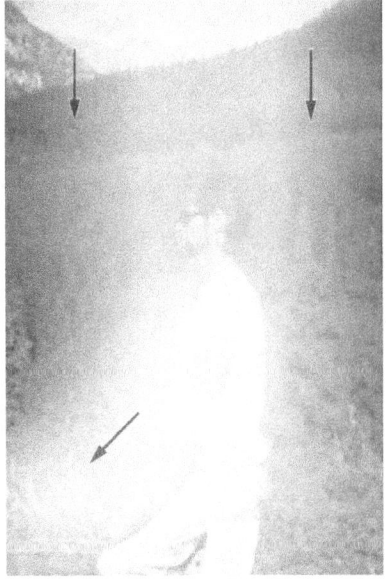

Figure 49: Shows sitting with crossed legs on a kneeling stool. On the right shows a variation of Conducting Heaven.

CHAPTER 16
FROM HANDS AND KNEES

Asanas from Hands and Knees are a great way to warm up the spine and shoulders. Common examples are Cat, Cow, Side Cow, Hip Circles, Hip Rocking, Arm and Leg Lifts with or without bringing knee to chest, Twists, Thread the Needle, Child's Pose and more.

Details on Threading the Needle

Threading the Needle starts from Hands and Knees by sliding one arm under your torso, reaching straight across (figure 50). Variations can include reaching above your head and reaching your arm pit to your opposite knee (figure 50).

Moving between these different positions, slowly, can be considered a Dynamic Variation, which can lead you to find a muscle(s) that need more attention than the others and alignments that work best for doing so. Dynamic Variations need to be done slowly until these areas are fully explored and then, if you choose, a Static Variation can be used for a more direct focusing. Remember that chronically tight areas will benefit greatly from some rubbing, movement and PE after being focused upon.

The position of your shoulder maters as well. If you reach your shoulder towards your hips, you will stretch your neck more. When it is closer to your ear, it will get deeper into the back of your shoulder. I recommend doing both. The neck is a very important area to keep relaxed for posture, as well as optimal blood and nervous system circulation. A relaxed neck can also make it easier to have a comfortable and deep night's sleep.

To intensify the stretching of your shoulder, place your non-reaching hand on your reaching one to hold it in place as you pull away with your torso. Be mindful of your limitations.

You can raise your non-reaching hand straight up and back to create a twist, which will require you to draw upon more core strength. Pushing your chest out intensifies this even more. Turning your head to look at your raised hand and pulling your shoulders back will help open your chest.

The position of your hips is also important. Try to keep them in their original position or reach them in the opposite direction your lower arm is reaching. You can also carefully explore their range as a Dynamic Variation.

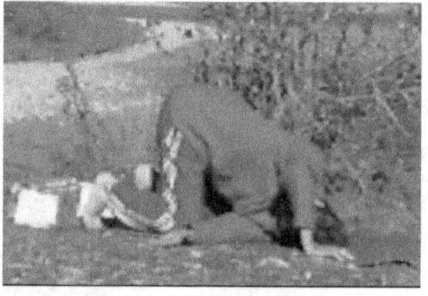

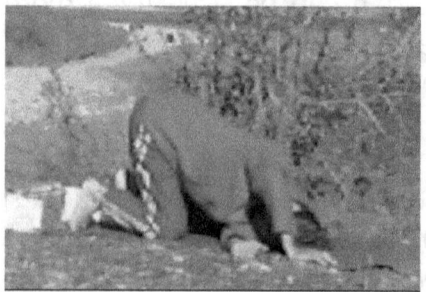
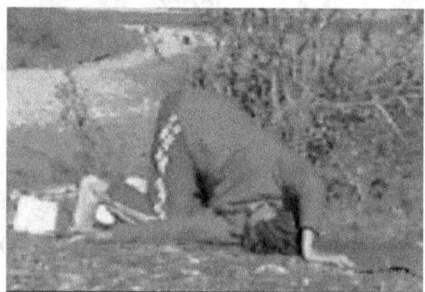

Figure 50: Shows the three standard arm positions for thread the needle.

As you progress with these variations, another modification can be included that will help find tight areas between your shoulder blades. This is an important area for people who carry stress there. It uses the same three hand positions with the opposite leg now reaching towards your head (figure 51). In general, the closer to your head you can get with your leg, the deeper into the asana you will be, but sometimes there will be position before this upper limit that will be important to explore.

You can explore these positions as a Dynamic Variation with your leg raised. It will challenge your core muscles, especially if you are reaching with your leg.

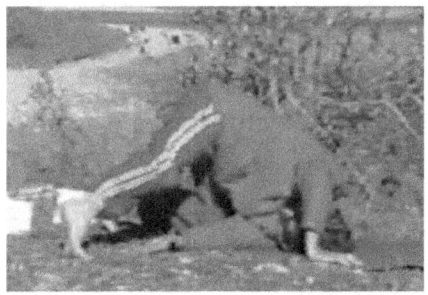

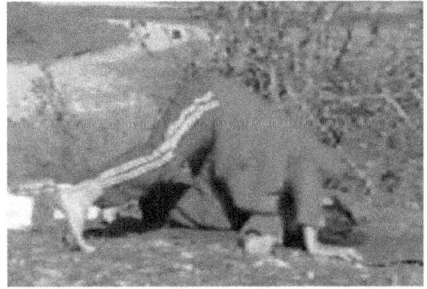 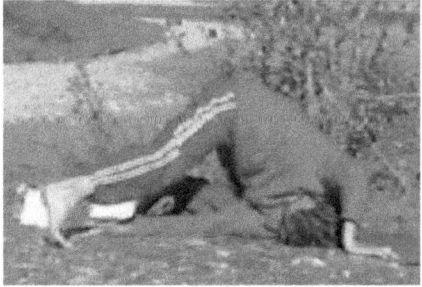

Figure 51: Moving your leg towards your head as you lean into your back can help focus the stretch up more of your mid-back.

This version of Thread the Needle, especially the dynamic variation form, is more challenging to balance and balance is very important, especially for heavier people. If you fall in this asana incorrectly, especially when there is a chronically tight area(s) involved, you could strain your back. Be mindful and cautious.

Finish by returning to Hands and Knees and doing some Cat, Cow and similar movements to help with circulation and realigning of your back and neck.

Details on Head Charging

When in Hands and Knees, it is very natural to hold your head in various ways to channel PE into it. Your brain is an extremely active and important part of your body. Physically it is estimated to burn 80% of an average person's calories. In regards to PE, it is constantly being influenced by them and trying to sense them (extrasensory perception/intuition). By charging it regularly, its health and performance will increase, giving you many benefits[90].

When you charge your brain regularly with the intent of enhancing its health and performance in a way that helps you live to your fullest potential, you do this. Your brain is a tool for your soul to program to help you live to your fullest potential. Charging your head helps it/you do this.

Charging your face with healthy PE is important as well. You express a lot of PE through your face. By helping to release unhealthy patterns from it and empower health ones, it becomes more natural for your expressions to be healthy.

---

[90] Head charging is discussed in more detail within *The Psychic Anatomy Exercises, Inner and Outer Success* and *Becoming Super Human.*

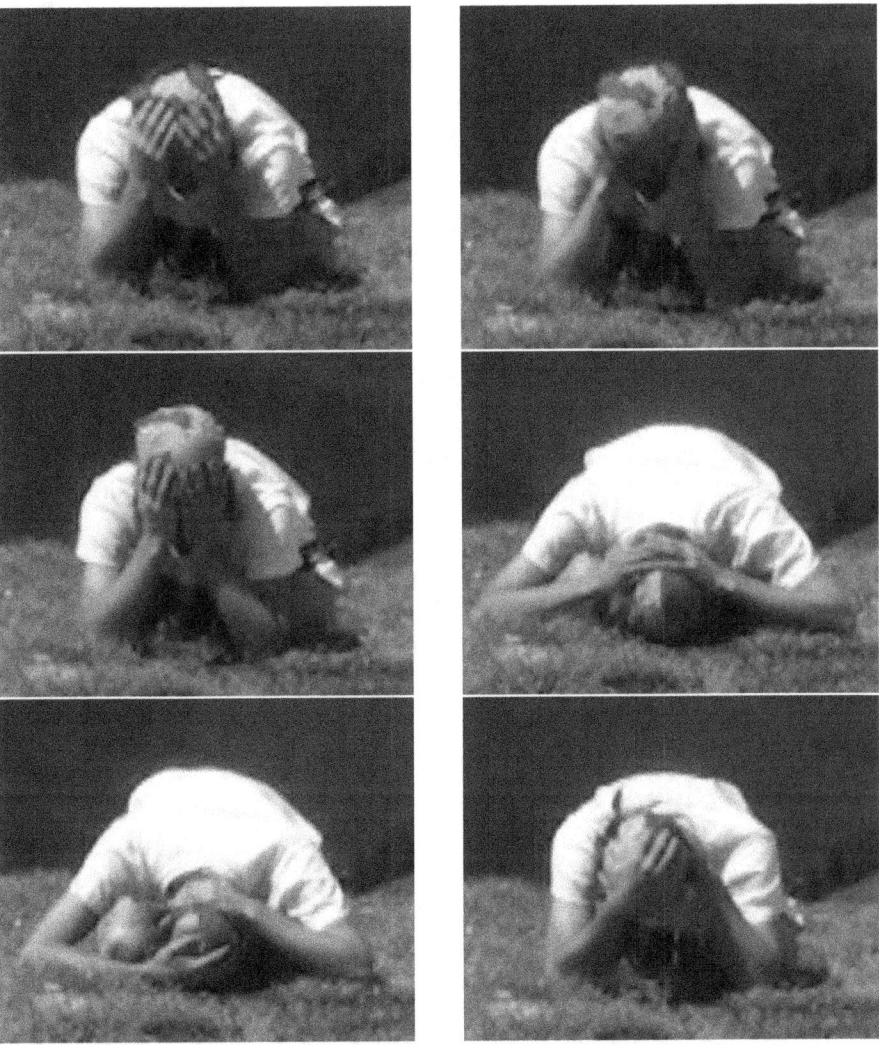

Figure 52: From top to bottom right. Part a shows charging the frontal cortex, which is important for working with memories, problem solving, controlling emotions and more. It is natural to grasp this part of the head when burdened with decisions. Part b shows charging the ears. Your ears listen for signals and take in a lot of information. Channeling healthy PE into them can be very relieving. Part c shows the charging of the face. It is natural to hold the face when emotional overwhelmed or embarrassed. Part d shows the charging of the back of the head, which is where a lot of sensory information in processed as well of coordinating your body. Parts e and f show positions for stabilizing/empowering the PE within your entire brain.

Details on Crow

Crow can be very challenging on a person's wrists. This does not have to be so. Your forearms should never project over your wrists. Bend your elbows so your forearms are perpendicular to the ground or behind your wrists. This will challenge your shoulders and core a lot more, which is what you want.

It helps to position your hands to have equal pressure on both sides of your palms. To make it even easier, keep your feet on the ground and bend your spine to slowly take your weight forward, lifting one leg at a time until you are ready to lift both.

If these suggestions are not enough, try putting a towel or Wrist Block under the back of your palms to raise your wrist off the ground, distributing more weight forward on your hands. Appendix H shows how to build a Wrist Block.

Details on Child's Pose

Child's Pose is intended to be a resting posture. Having your arms by your side and completely releasing your body into relaxation is key. This can greatly help relieve fresh tension from over-doing asanas. Focusing on strained area(s) or your entire body as expanding and contracting with your breath can help improve circulation of fluids of PE. When you intend for healthy PE (aka. prana) to be breathed by specific parts of your body and the entire body, this happens[91] and the healthy PE will help them/it recover.

Child's Pose can also be used to help open the back. Reaching out of your hip with your arms while tightening your core greatly helps open your lower back. Adding a twist can take it even deeper as well as include more of your hip muscles (figure

---

[91] Maybe not intensely at first, but I time you will get more powerful.

53). Twisting with a reaching arm raised, with or without a tight core, can help open your entire back, especially the areas that are tighter than the rest.

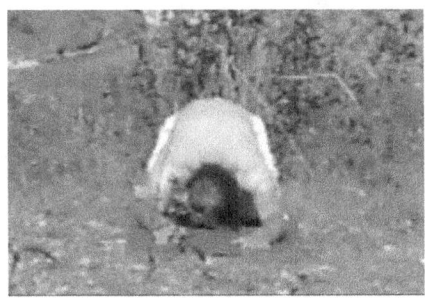 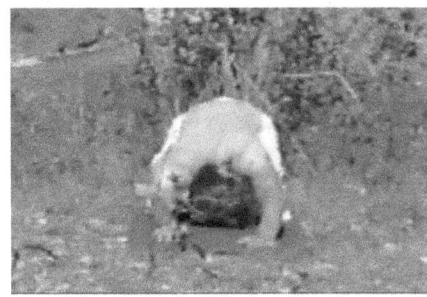

Figure 53: Shows regular Child's Pose on the left and with a twist on the right.

These twists can also engage you ribs as you breathe. Be careful here, ribs can be easily strained. Test your limits slowly.

General Alignment, Experiential Meditation and focusing on balancing and harmonizing psychic anatomy can be done in Child's Pose. When in Child's Pose, you are resting, which makes it easier to check in with yourself, recenter, balance, harmonize and recharge if necessary.

CHAPTER 17
FROM STANDING ON KNEES

Standing on Knees is a great position for most of the psychic energy exercises in Part 1. A General Alignment can be done quickly, bringing more balance and harmony to yourself. Yin-Yang and Sine Wave are quick to do as well, giving you a chance to focus on balancing a harmonizing your aura and/or hara.

Many people find it difficult to stay comfortably standing on their knees for spending longer periods of time doing these exercises. Luckily, it is very easy to lower into kneeling on your heels[92] or a kneeling stool, making it easier to spend more time doing them comfortably.

If you have been still for a significant length of time. Move into asanas slowly to avoid head rushes, lack of coordination and balance. Doing a few easier asanas to awaken your body and get more grounded before challenging yourself physically is recommended. If you think you got a bit stiff from being still, I recommend a few easier asanas as well (ex. those from Hands and Knees).

Details on Half Swimmer and Mountain Climber

From Standing on Knees, lean over to one side and place the hand under your shoulder on the ground as you wave your other hand up and over your head till it is reaching above your head towards your soul gates to enter Half Swimmer. You can also reach back a bit to open your chest. Your knee on the ground should be slightly off center with your hip, towards your

---

[92] Only if it can be done without feeling strain during and after doing so.

other foot. This will help to avoid hip strain. This is even more important when you lift your other leg off the ground to challenge your core muscles (figure 54).

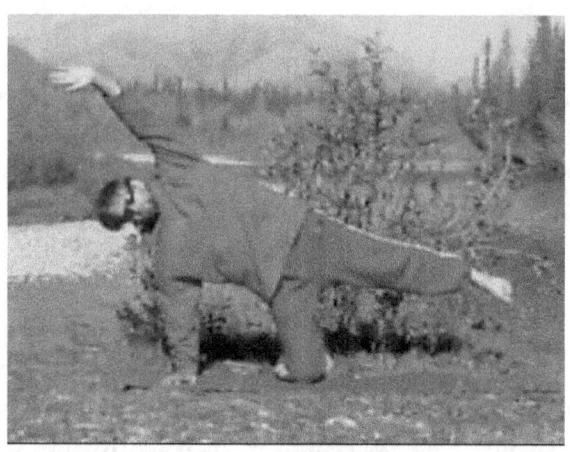

Figure 54: Half Swimmer with one leg lifted. This challenges your core muscles more. By moving your lifted leg back and forth, up and down, with or without your reaching arm moving forth and back, down and up or back and forth, up and down, will challenge your core muscles even more. Be mindful that your knee on the ground is slightly of center with your hip, towards your lifted foot to avoid unhealthy strain on your hip.

With one leg lifted, you can move your lifted leg back and forth, up and down, with or without your reaching arm moving forth and back, down and up or back and forth, up and down, will challenge your core muscles even more. Be mindful that your knee on the ground is slightly of center with your hip, towards your lifted foot to avoid hip strain.

Be mindful not to push your self too hard with these movements before you are ready, because there are many small muscles involved that could get strained. Be mindful.

From this position (figure 55a), there are several options.

Option 1

When returning to Standing on Knees, Sweep your raised hand up and over your head and continuing Sweeping until it is at the bottom of your reach, with your palm facing up towards your seventh chakra. Sweep your other hand off the ground till it is at the top of your reach, with your palm facing down towards your first chakra (figure 55f). You are now in Yin-Yang (discussed in Chapter 4). Focus on there being balance and harmony within your chakra system and psychic anatomy in general. As you make these movements, pull your extended leg in so you are Standing on Knees when you enter Yin-Yang.

You can also simply sweep your reaching hand to be the top of Yin-Yang and your lower hand to be the bottom. This movement is more peaceful, letting you stay in a place of stillness more easily, while the previous causes more PE to move (Sweeping). They both have their advantages depending on your state of being.

In both movements, you can move into Sine Wave instead as well.

Options 2

Sweep your reaching hand up and over until you are in Mountain Climber (figure 55e). Mountain Climber can also be entered at the end of Option 1.

Options 3

This is my favorite option. Figures 55 shows it from Half Swimmer to Mountain Climber, but it can also be done from Mountain Climber to Half Swimmer. From Half Swimmer draw a circle with your reaching arm in front of you ending at your reaching leg. From there or slightly before, start bringing your arm that is on the ground towards it and then up into Mountain Climber.

From Mountain Climber, you can enter Yin-Yang/Sine Wave as discussed in Option 1 or do Option 3 in reverse.

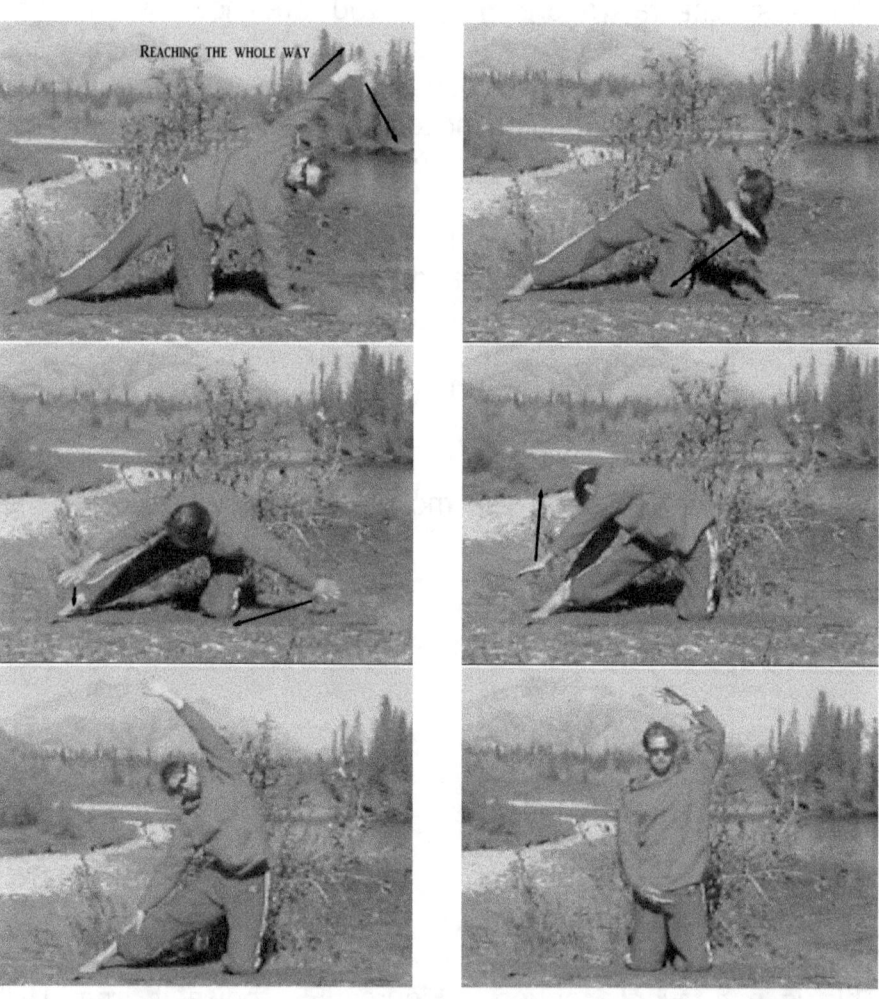

Figure 55: Part a top left, part f bottom right. See Option 3 for a discussion on the Dynamic Variation of Half Swimmer to Mountain Climber.

Option 3 is a great Dynamic Variation that can help find key muscles the need more attention (ex. a Static Variation, rubbing, focusing healthy PE). By giving these areas extra attention, a big difference can be noticed to the comfort and quality of your posture. Be mindful though, always be mindful, because there are several smaller muscles that could get strained if you loose your balance.

CHAPTER 18
FROM FORWARD FOLD

As you approach the limits of your flexibility in Forward Fold, try to rotate your pelvis so there is an arch in your lower back. This arch is hard to obtain for most people, but the effort of doing so is what you are looking for.

You can see this arch in Halfway Lift on the left of figure 56, while in Forward Fold there is a lot more curvature (right). Just by gently contracting the muscles that pull you in the direction on this arch. It will strengthen your lower back as it improves the quality of the stretch. This can over exert your lower back muscles if you try too hard, so be mindful.

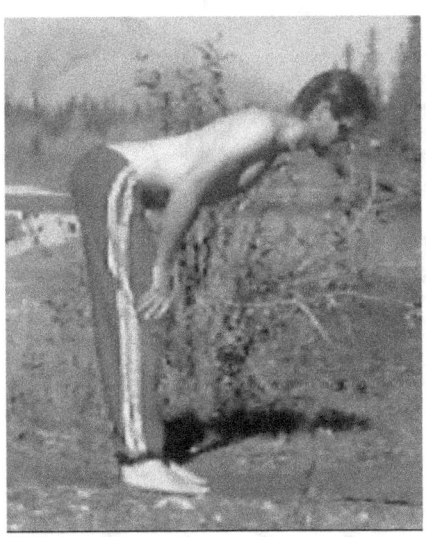 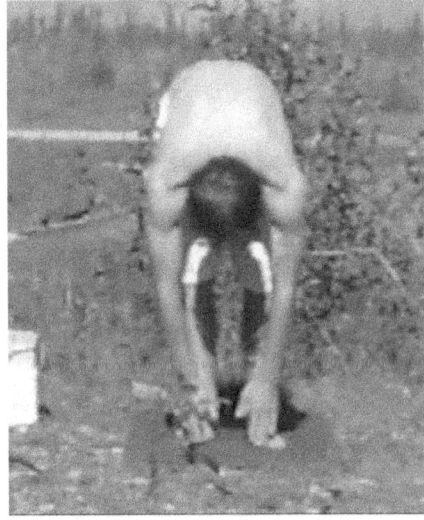

Figure 56: Shows the lower back arch in Halfway Lift and Forward Fold (sort of).

Using the Kneeling Stool described in Appendix H or the seat of a chair to push into with your hands can help with creating this arch. I show an example of this in Chapter 21.

Most of the variations discussed in Chapter 14 can be applied while in Forward Fold, such as twist, etc.

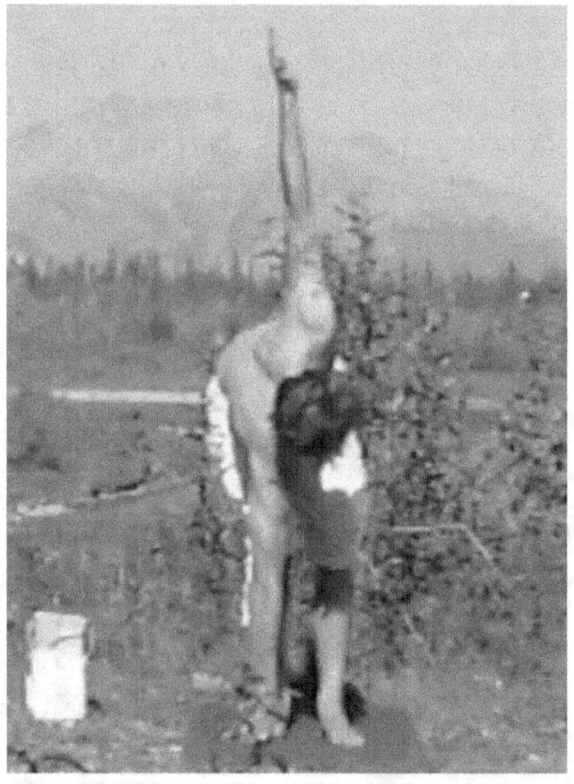

Figure 57: Twist in Forward Fold is a great way keep the spine flexible. It requires the muscles that are being twisted to support the weight of your body, which can greatly help develop their strength.

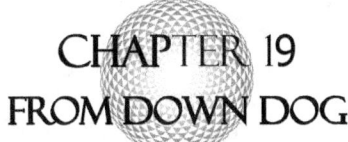

CHAPTER 19
FROM DOWN DOG

Many Dynamic and Static Variations can be done in Down Dog. Three Legged Dog is an excellent example of this. Just twisting your hips, leaning to each side, tracing circle with your tail bone and more are other options work well. Remember that Dynamic and Static Variations can help you find tension in your body, but they can also help create it if done over aggressively. Be patient and mindful as you explore them.

In Chapter 14 I discussed pulling your spine to the center of your body. Down Dog is a great time to practice this. Remember to mindfully try to keep an arch in your lower back as you do.

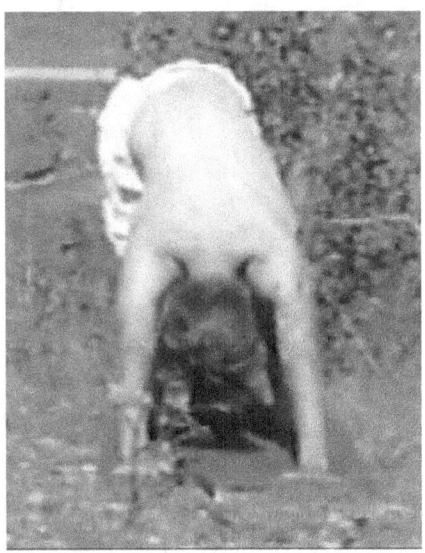 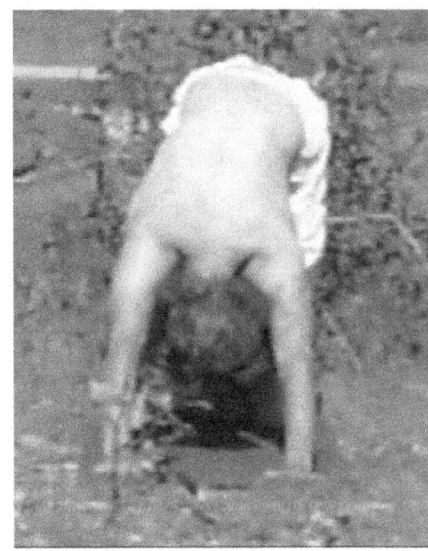

Figure 58: Hip lean in Down Dog

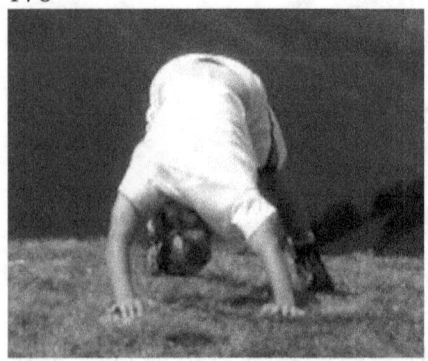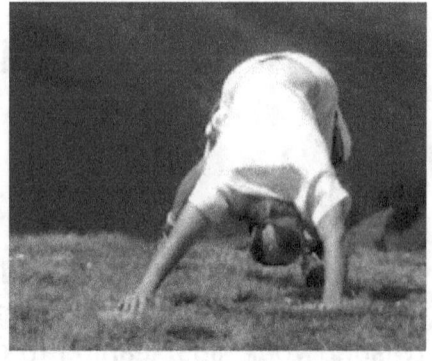

Figure 59: Full body lean in Down Dog

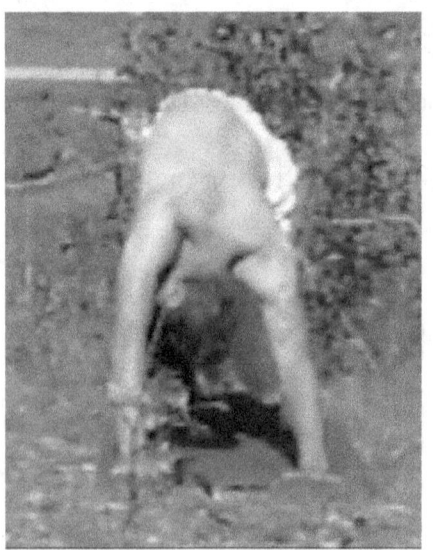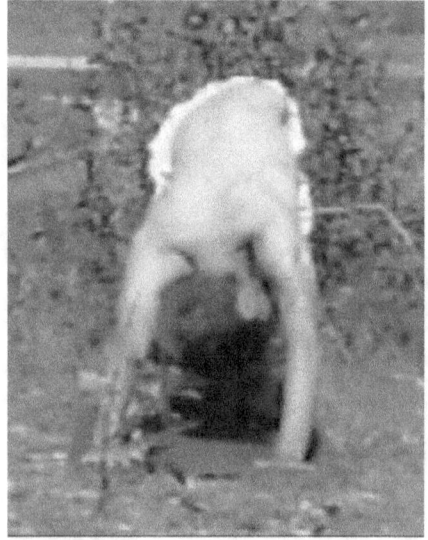

Figure 60: Twist in Down Dog

Down Dog can be a resting pose once your flexibility allows for it to be so. This is a great time to check in and do some balancing and harmonizing. Embracing Earth is another great option, because it will help ground, rejuvenate and empower you physically for the rest of your practice (figure 61).

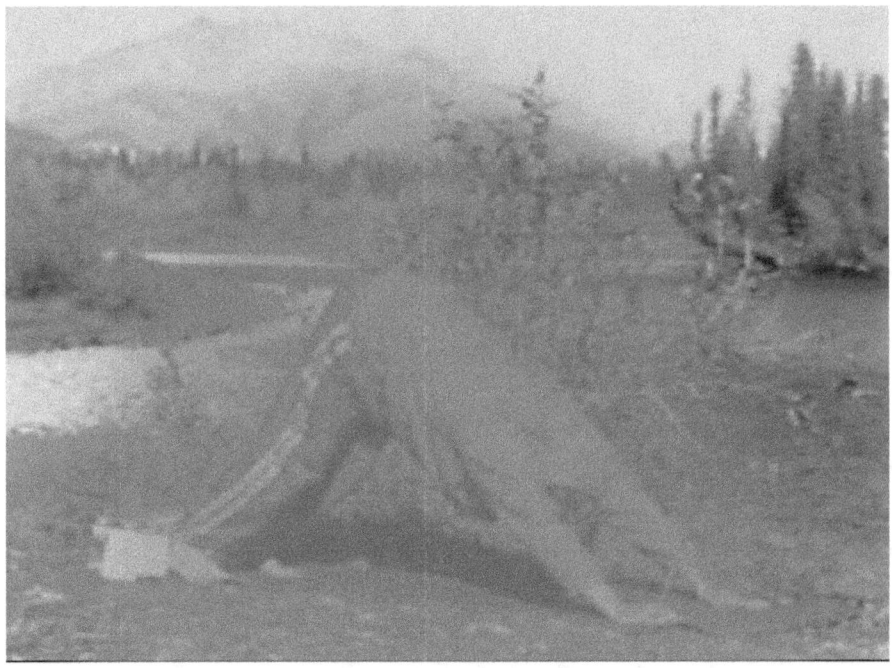

Figure 61: Embracing Earth in Down Dog.

Details on Plank

Plank is one of those wonderful asanas that can be included many times in your practice. When in Plank lengthen your spine, reach with your head and heels and create a straight line between your heels and head (figure 57). This will help develop your core muscles, but only for a little while, then you need to modify it for more development[93]. There are several options for doing this.

---

[93] Core muscles are very important for most movements and postures.

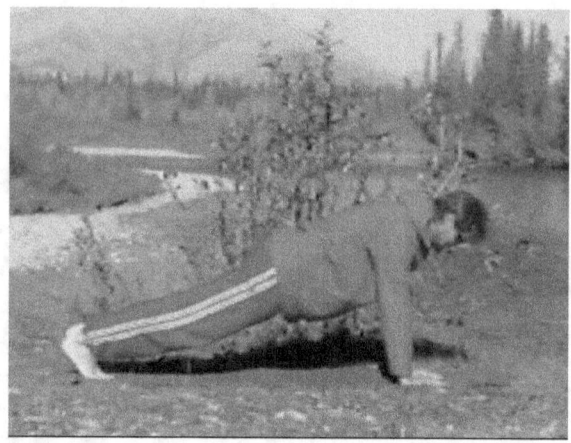

Figure 57: When in Plank, lift out of your hips, reach with your head and heels, creating a straight line between your heels and head.

Option 1

Try swaying left to right as shown in figure 58. You can also include your hips right to left or left to right as well. Another option is tracing circles with your shoulders and/or hips.

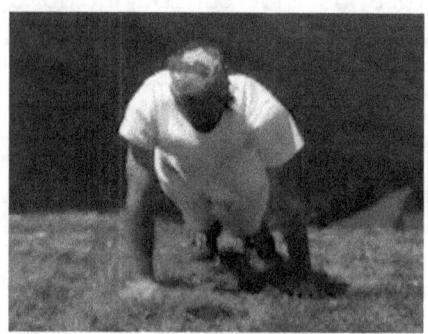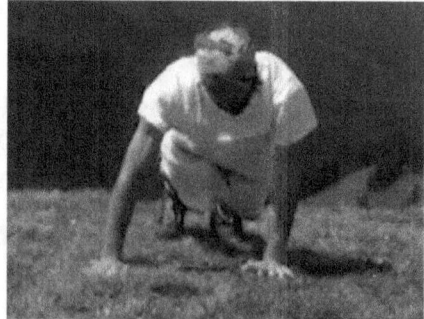

Figure 58: Shows swaying while in Plank. Remember that you can include your hips.

Option 2

If you sway far enough, you can sway into Side Plank. Small swaying motions can be done here as well, but I only recommend small movements, because your shoulder is under a lot more pressure and balancing is more challenging.

Option 3

Option 3 applies to regular Plank and Side Plank. It is the lifting of a leg and/or arm as shown in figure 59. To make this even more challenging, try making it into a Dynamic Variation by moving your lifted limb(s) front to back, up and down or in circles. For example move your leg front to back while moving your arm back to front or front to back.

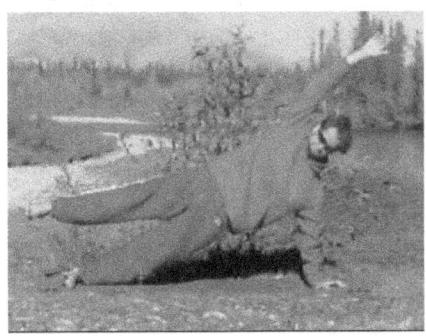 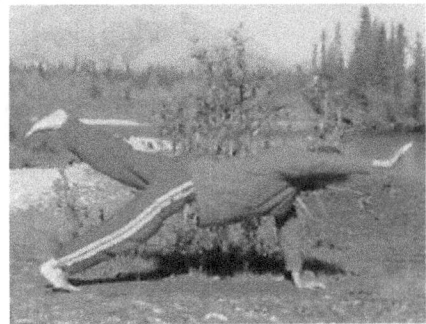

Figure 59: Variations of Plank and Side Plank.

If any of these options are hard on your wrists, you can use Wrist/Ankle Blocks (Appendix H) or a towel to raise your wrist to distribute more weight upon upon the ball of your hands and fingers.

Details on Pigeon

Pigeon is one of those asanas that people tend have a love-hate relationship with; usually with the people that need it the most. Pigeon targets lengthening the hip-tensors, which can be uncomfortable if hip tensors are tight. Well worth the discomfort, because of the relief it can bring to lower back discomforts. I highly recommend incorporating it in your practice daily.

Pigeon is usually held a bit longer than other asanas. This is a great time to do some reflexology on your feet and/or hands. A bit of foot and/or hand reflexology can really optimize the natural flow of PE threw them, helping your entire physical body as well[94].

In the morning and before going to bed is a great time to do this asana, as well as other basic asanas. Even just 5 minutes a day of moving through a few basic asanas can make a big difference to the health and performance of your physical body and more physical parts of your psychic anatomy.

---

[94] I discuss Reflexology in *The Psychic Energy Reality*.

CHAPTER 20
FROM STANDING

Standing is an excellent position for doing all the psychic energy exercises in Part 1 for long periods of time. From Standing, it is easy to sit in a chair and get out of one without disturbing the alignment of your spine or meditative state much, which is a great for when you feel drawn to go deeper into what you are doing and/or giving your legs a break. Kneeling stools are options as well, but can be more disruptive compared to a chair.

Standing Twists are excellent movements to bring relief to the back when Standing for long periods of time. Remember to keep your spine straight when you do, this will minimize disruption within your psychic anatomy. PE can move more easily and precisely when the spine is straight and still. This is very beneficial when Conducting and to a lesser degree when Embracing Heaven and/or Earth.

Figure 60: Standing Twists

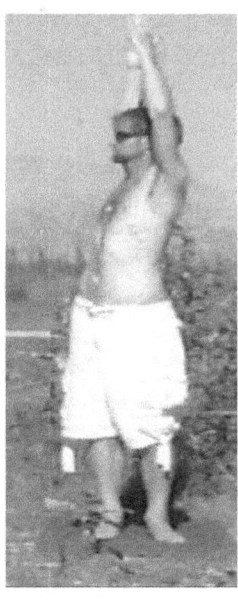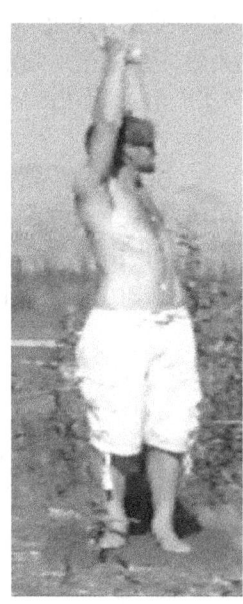

It is common to sweep arms up wide when entering and leaving Standing. These arm movements are very similar to movements in Qi-gong, which are used to move and spread healthy PE in your auric bodies. Some forms of Yoga also teach this concept (ex. Tantra and Kundalini practices).

It is less common for Yoga practices to teach keeping hands in close as they are lifted and lowered. When doing these movements, you are essentially practicing the most common type of Qi-gong movement, which is called Scanning in Psychic Anatomy Yoga (see Chapter 2).

These movements will often result in your intuition guiding you to focus health PE upon specific parts. Trust it. Your intuition is always right. There will be times when it might seem like it is not, but if you stay mindful and *accept the outcome*, you'll likely see how it was in time.

Sometimes your Extrasensory Perception (ESP) will become aware of differences as you Scan over your body. These sensations will become more revealing as you develop your awareness of PE. Awareness of PE can help greatly help optimize the health and performance of your psychic anatomy, as well as help you help others optimize theirs. Energy healing and Psychic Anatomy Treatments are discussed in *Psychic Anatomy Treatments.*

I recommend these movements (Scanning) to help kick start your intuition/ESP, especially in the beginning. With practice, you will find yourself flowing into and out of exercises naturally. Still, Scanning can is a good technique for circulating PE.

These movements are discussed in more detail below.

Details on Moving into/out of Standing from/to Forward Fold

When you are in Forward Fold, focus your attention on connecting to Earth PE that resonates with the healthy PE already in your psychic anatomy. Imagine these Earth PE spiraling counter-clockwise beneath your feet. When you are ready, raise them up on an inhalation as the counter-clockwise spiral forms into a column of healthy Earth PE that you Embrace or Conduct threw your psychic anatomy and around you. This can be done with raising your arms spread wide, held in close or somewhere in between. It is common to take your hands all the way up to be reaching above your head.

After Embracing or Conducting Earth, you can start Ascending[95] them or focusing them threw specific systems of your psychic anatomy (ex. meridians, aura, hara). You want to wait until you have establish the Earth Exercise in a general way to avoid sending too much power or disharmony threw these systems. By waiting, you give yourself an extra second or so, which is enough to harmonize with the energies and open these parts of your psychic anatomy up to the Earth PE under more control.

The Extraordinary Vessel Exercise and ida of the Sushuma Exercise are particularly good for this, because they naturally draw upon Earth PE to empower your internal aura. Both exercises are discussed in Chapter 3.

Option 1

With both hands above your head you can greatly empower your connection to Heaven. You can continue to Embrace or Conduct Earth as you do this. As you do, start building a clockwise spiral of healthy Heaven PE above your head[96].

---

[95]   Ascending discussed in Chapter 11 .

[96]   This spiral is in the opposite direction as the one beneath your feet. Counter-clockwise means PE are flowing towards you.

From here lower both hands, palms facing your center as in Scanning till they are at the bottom of your reach, focusing the column of healthy Heaven PE threw you and down your legs, into the Earth as you enter Forward Fold. You can also do this with arms spread wide, spreading the healthy PE around you and/or pushing away unhealthy PE. Somewhere in between is fine as well. Be mindful and do what comes naturally.

Option 2

Do some Scanning with hands held in or arms spread wide a few times before returning to Forward Fold. Keeping your hands close, palms facing your center, is good for circulating and releasing PE within you (ex. internal aura, chakras, hara, etc.), while arm spread wide is better for spreading and circulating these healthy PE and releasing unhealthy PE around you (auric bodies). The flow of Heaven and Earth PE will help empower the healthy PE and carry away the unhealthy ones. Remember to have the intention for these released unhealthy PE to be recycled by the Earth and/or vegetation.

It is very common for your intuition to guide you to focus on specific areas or move into specific exercises when Scanning; your ESP can play a significant role in this as it develops.

Yin-Yang and Sine Wave are common exercises to incorporate during these movements as well. Remember to alternate hand positions in conjunction with asana flows for left and right sides of the body.

You can carry on from here with Options 1, 3 or 4.

Option 3

After Embracing or Conducting Heaven, you can start Descending[97] them or focusing them threw specific systems of your psychic anatomy (ex. hara, aura, meridians). You may want to wait until you have establish the Heaven Exercise to avoid sending too much power or disharmony threw these systems. By waiting, you also give yourself an extra second or so, which is enough to harmonize with the energies and open these parts of your psychic anatomy up to the Heaven PE under more control.

The soul gates of the Turning Inwards exercise and pingala of the Sushuma Exercise are particularly good for this, because they naturally draw upon Heaven PE to empower you. These exercises is discussed in Chapters 5 and 11 .

You can carry on from here with Options 1, 2 or 4.

Option 4

With both hands above your head, you can focus health Earth PE or PE in general upon your Soul Gates, which might result in them shining PE upon you. From here you can Descend through your psychic anatomy step by step or intuitively (only focusing on specific areas). I recommend that you Embrace or Conduct Heaven as you do this, but sometimes it will be best to wait till you have Descended at least once first. When ready return to Forward Fold as described in Option 1.

You can carry on from here with Options 1, 2 or 3.

---

[97] Ascending discussed in Chapter 11.

Details on Leaning Backward (Back Bend)

From Standing, lean backward, stretching the front of your body, opening up your conception vessel and front chakras. Doing this requires some good core strength to protect your spine. Try moving the pressure on your spine up and down.

Return to Standing and then go into Forward Fold, while being mindful of your lower back as you try to lengthen your spine opening up your governing vessel and back chakras. Rounding your spine is an option. Spend sometime feeling your vessels and chakras in these different positions.

Details on Balancing Asanas

I've been in a lot of classes that move from one balancing asana to another on the same leg. It has been my experience that most people need a break in-between, so blood can flow threw their leg again. Please make time for yourself if you feel you need to create movement in a part of your body that has been under tension. Straining a part of your body with insufficient blood supply has no benefits to my knowledge.

Balancing asanas can get easy after awhile. Incorporating some movements can really enhance how they challenge you. See Chapter 19 for examples of movements in Plank and Side Plank.

Details on Eagle

Eagle is an excellent asana to do Heaven and Earth Exercises in, especially near the end.

When you finish with Eagle, let the restricted PE from the crossing and squeezing of your arms and legs rush threw you as and burst out as your arms sweep up and out and your lifted leg returns to the ground (figure 61). Intend for unhealthy PE to be pushed out and way into the Earth and vegetation for recycling. Also intend for healthy PE to be spread around you as your psychic anatomy, specifically your auric bodies, expand.

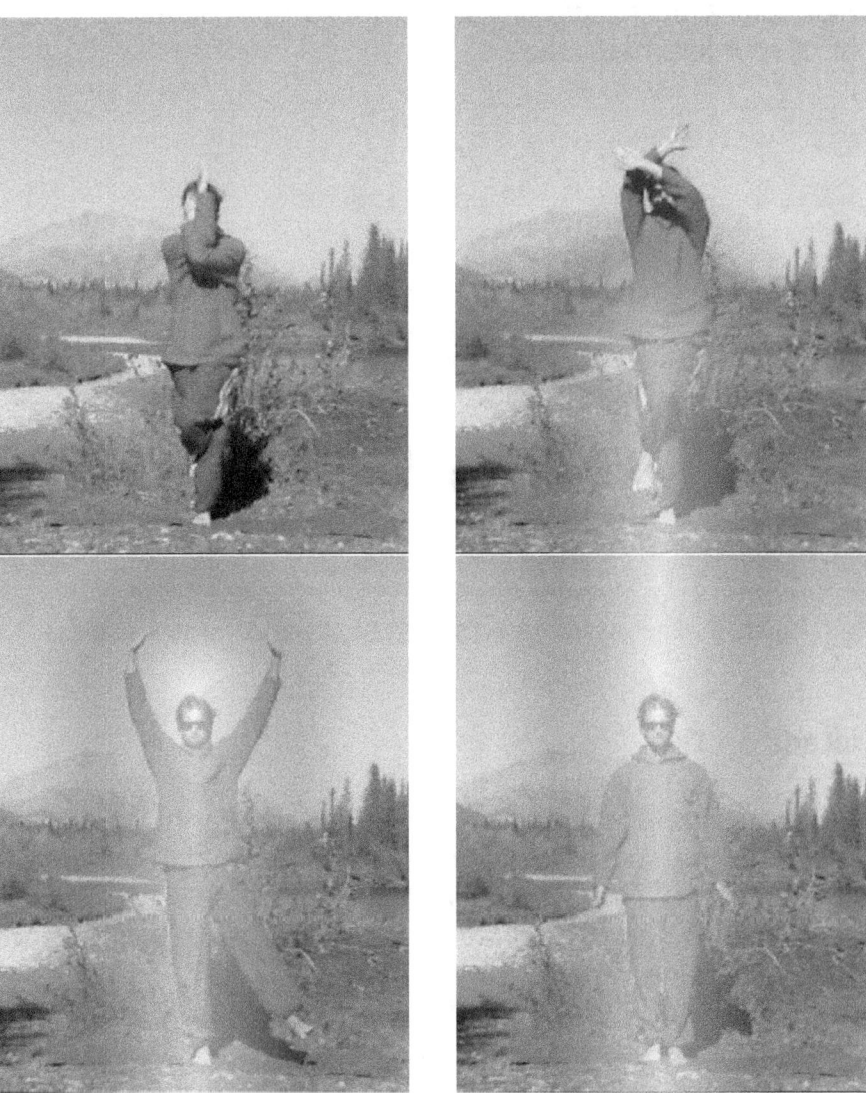

Figure 61: Burst out of Eagle, sending a burst of healthy Earth PE threw you and continue Conducting them in Standing.

When the additional leg returns to the ground, you can empower your flow of Earth[98] and/or Heaven PE to help flush and empower you with. A great set of options to explore.

Wrist stretched can also be done when in Eagle (figure 62). Wrist, similar to hands, are important to the flow of PE in and out of your internal aura.

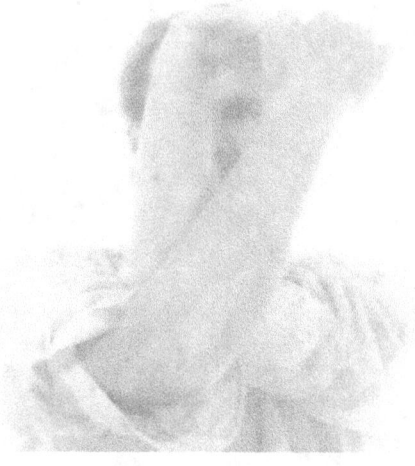

Figure 62: Shows how the wrists can be stretched while in Eagle.

Details on Tree

Tree is an excellent asana to do Heaven and Earth Exercises in for different reasons. Your arms are free to move, which makes all the psychic energy exercises and General Techniques in general easy to do. The movements will challenge your balance which is an added bonus.

I like to I focus on facilitating balance and harmony in my aura with Yin-Yang and hara with Sine Wave. Interchanging hand positions before leaving Tree.

---

[98]   Assuming you are not already doing so.

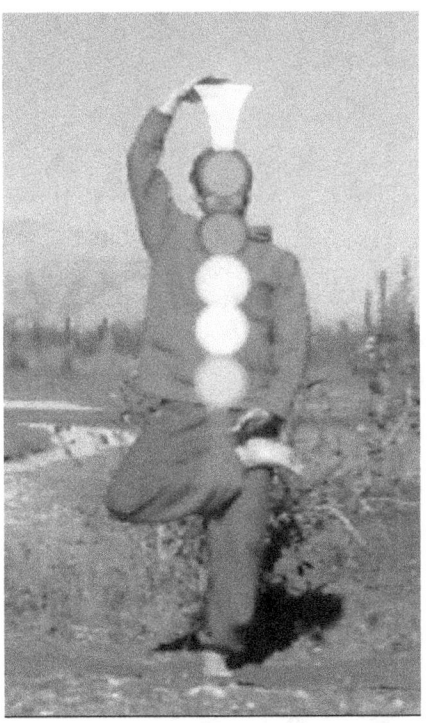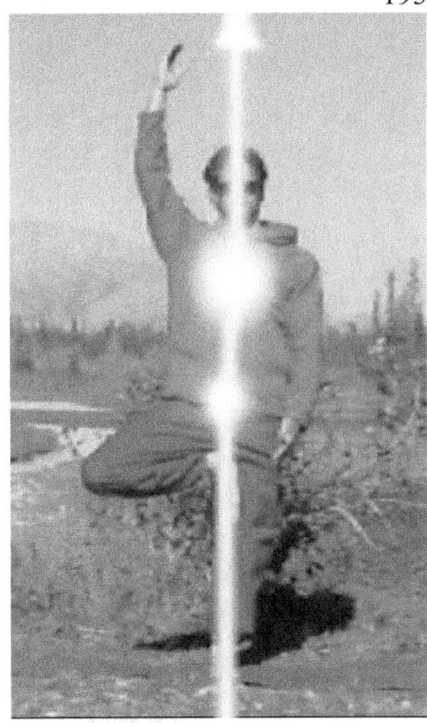

Figure 63: Yin-Yang on left, Sine Wave on right.

You can also do some reflexology on yourself when in Half-Lotus (figure 64). A bit of hand and/or foot reflexology can really optimize the natural flow of PE threw them, helping the entire physical body as well.

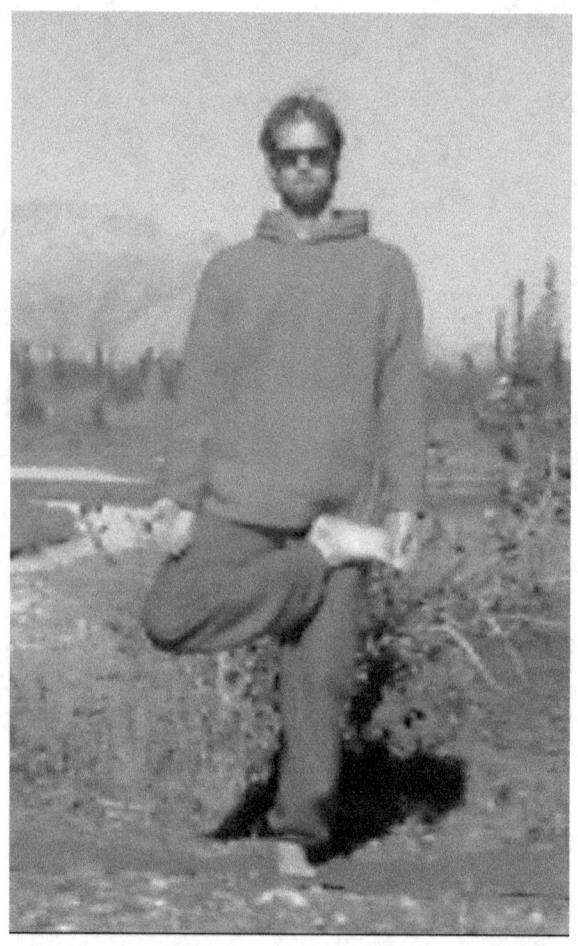

Figure 64: Doing some reflexology in Tree with Half-Lotus.

CHAPTER 21
FROM STRADDLED STANDING

While in these asanas, your core and legs can be strengthened by lifting and lower your hips. This will also help find any muscles that are tighter than those around them. If you are doing so, you can pump PE up from the Earth into your psychic anatomy and physical body[99] at the same time. You can also include or do on their own, Dynamic Variations, such as rocking your hips back and forth, leans and twists to challenge your core muscles, coordination and balance more.

These movements are only to be practiced by those with strong core muscles, good coordination and balance, because they can strain the body if done improperly, which can be easy to do. If you do strain yourself during these movements or at any time, go into Child's Pose or an asana that is comfortable and lets you gently stretch and relax (pulse) the area strained as you focus healthy PE into and around it. This pulsing helps for flushing PE and blood in and out of the area, helping it recover. Sweeping away the unhealthy PE that are released during this process will help as well. Keep mindfully moving it periodically later on to keep helping fresh blood get in and strained blood get out.

Remember that PE are controlled by your attention. If you focus your attention on trying to "heal your injured hip", you'll be empowering PE associated with those emotions and thoughts "heal", "injured" and "hips"). Try not to include concepts like "injured", rather focus on "restoring health and performance", "rejuvenation", etc.

---

[99]   Note that bringing PE into your physical body is really bringing PE into your psychic anatomy, specifically your Internal Aura (Discussed in *The Psychic Energy Reality, The Psychic Anatomy Exercises* and in depth within *The Interface Between Psychic Energies and the Physical Body.*

Some Straddled Standing asanas can put excessive tension on the outside of your ankles. Foam blocks or Wrist/Ankle Blocks[100] can be used to lift the outside of your foot/feet up, reducing tension on the outside of your ankle. Sand naturally gives you this support and is usually in a beautiful environment for practicing in.

Straddled Standing asanas are commonly practiced by beginners with their abdomen fairly relaxed. Small bends in their knees and little reach coming out of their hips. This is fine, but as they/you develop in your practice, pulling your abdomen in and up as you reach out of your hips takes these asanas to a whole new level. The same goes with reaching with your arms and legs, holding them firm as you enter in and out of these asanas and their variations.

The final thing I will comment on before discussing PE aspects of these asanas, is pulling your spine to the center of your body and expanding out the front. Centering your spine was discussed in Chapter 14.

When moving between Straddled Standing asanas, be mindful of your head alignment, so you can keep a connection with Heaven as you flow. Even if you are not consciously connecting to Heaven, you might still be drawing PE from it. This does not mean you have to always maintain optimal head alignment. It just means be mindful of it in case it is a good idea. If it is and you miss it, its not a big deal, but if it is and you catch it, then it is a big deal, because you have moved forward.

As you advance in Psychic Anatomy Yoga, you will spend more time doing the psychic energy exercises of Part 1[101] in these asanas, flowing with your intuition into other exercises and asanas. When this starts to happen, it will become more important to lean into your back leg and press into it with your

---

[100] Discussed in Appendix H.
[101] As well as some from *The Psychic Anatomy Exercises.*

front leg to take weight of your front leg so you can stay in them longer. Remember to keep a micro-bend in your back leg to avoid knee joint strain (figure 65) and to be extra mindful of possible joint strain in general. You can also change your leg positions, such as straightening them, moving you hips about and other movements to bring relief to your physical body. Fatigue is often caused by poor circulation.

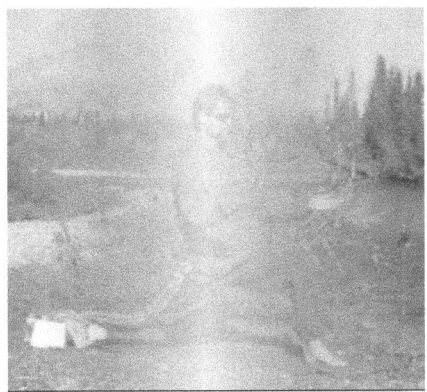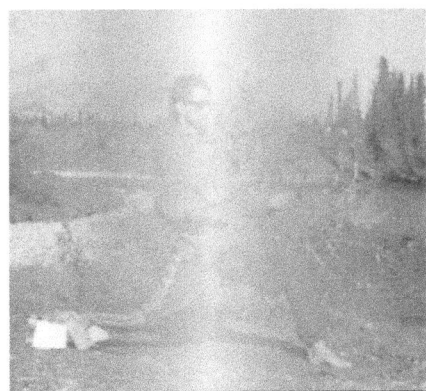

Figure 65: Two positions for Standing Lunge, not leaning into back leg (left) and leaning into back leg (right). Conducting Heaven and Earth is shown in both images.

Details on Warrior 2

Be centered in healthy PE at your heart chakra, project PE that serves your greatest good into your future with your front hand to help manifest and learn with. With your back hand project it into your past to help heal and learn from your past. This is a symbolic use of PE that acts on the less physical dimensions of reality[102].

---

[102] See *A Formula for Evolution* or *God's Journey* for a discussions on these dimensions.

Details on Standing Lunge

Place one or both hands on your thighs to help pull your spine out of your hips.

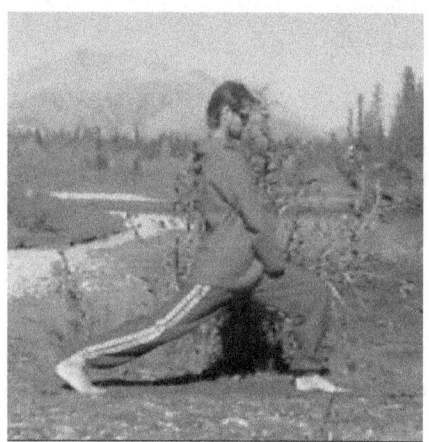
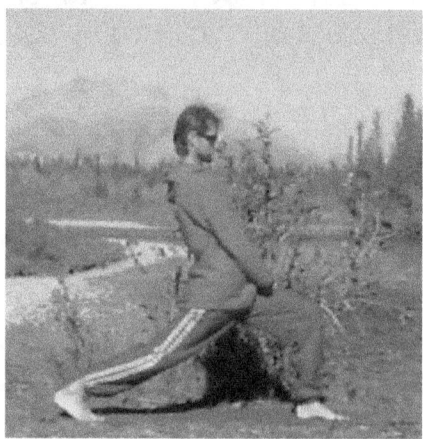

Figure 66: Using arms to help pull spine out of hips. Right side also shows leaning into back leg, which also stretches the stomach muscles when pulling them in.

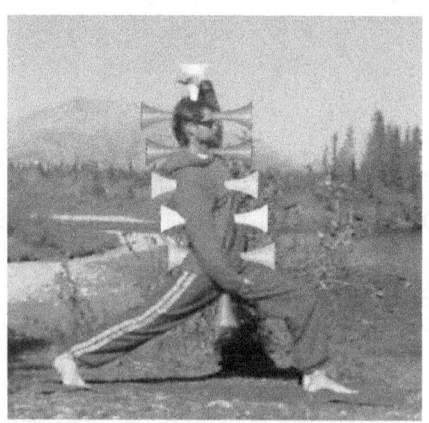
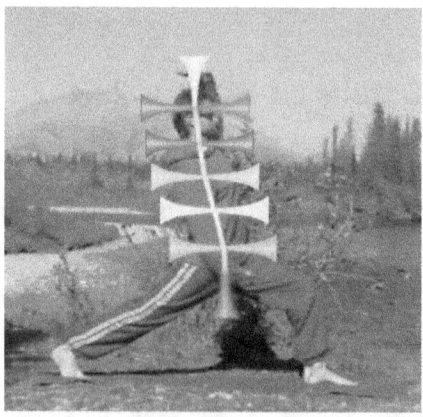

Figure 67: Shows Yin Yang on left with chakras only visible outside the body and chakras and chakra column visible inside and outside the body on the right. You can see there is a bit of a lean into the back leg as well.

Benefits of a Kneeling Stool/Support Blocks:

Kneeling Stools have been discussed as excellent tools for the psychic energy exercises of Part 1, during and after asana practices. The design I present in Appendix H is strong enough to be used as a support block in two positions as well (figure 68)[103].

Many asanas can be intense and challenging to balance in, especially in the beginning. This combination can result in strain, especially when balance is lost. There is no need to risk strain. Support blocks are inexpensive and easy to transport. Kneeling Stools are easy and inexpensive to make, are easy to transport and have other purposes as well.

The intensity and challenge to balance in these asanas encourages people to place a forearm on their knee or lower thigh to gain support. If you are working your core muscles and want to hover your forearm above or slightly on your thigh (not knee) for mild support when needed, this is OK, but not as a support. Too much pressure will block circulation, weakening starved muscles and ligaments and could cause cardiovascular problems in the area for some people.

---

[103] Angles brackets can greatly reinforce these Kneeling Stools; see Appendix H.

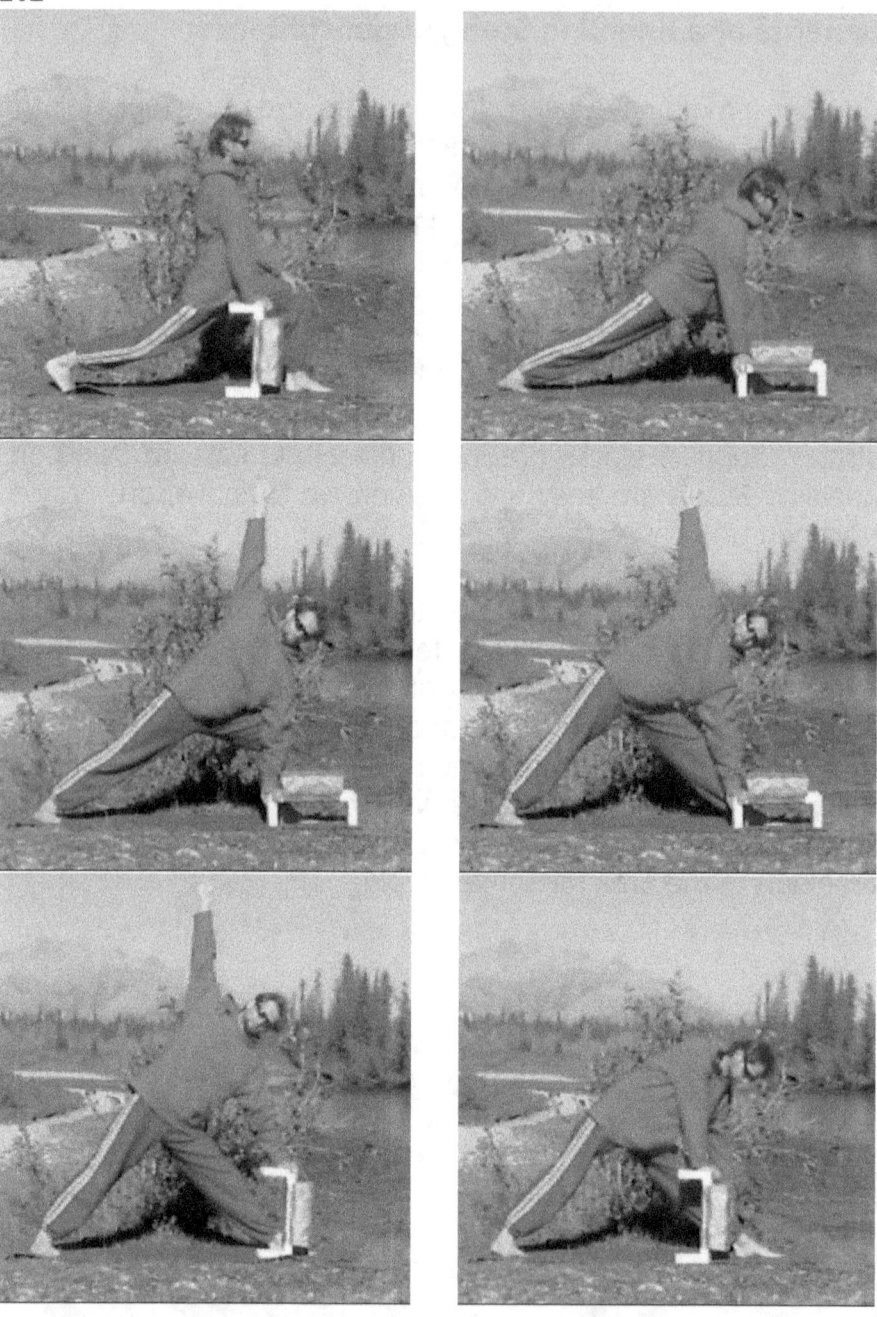

Figure 68: Use of the Kneeling Stool in Appendix H as a support block.

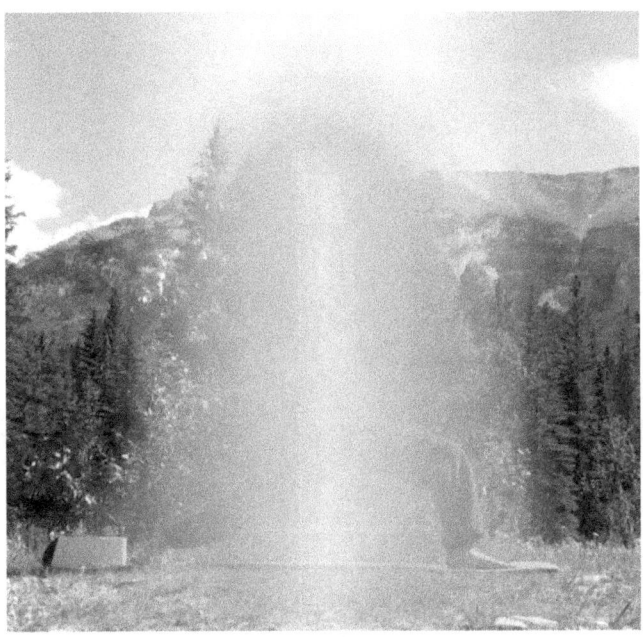

Figure 69: Shows Embracing Earth and Conducting Heaven in Warrior 1.

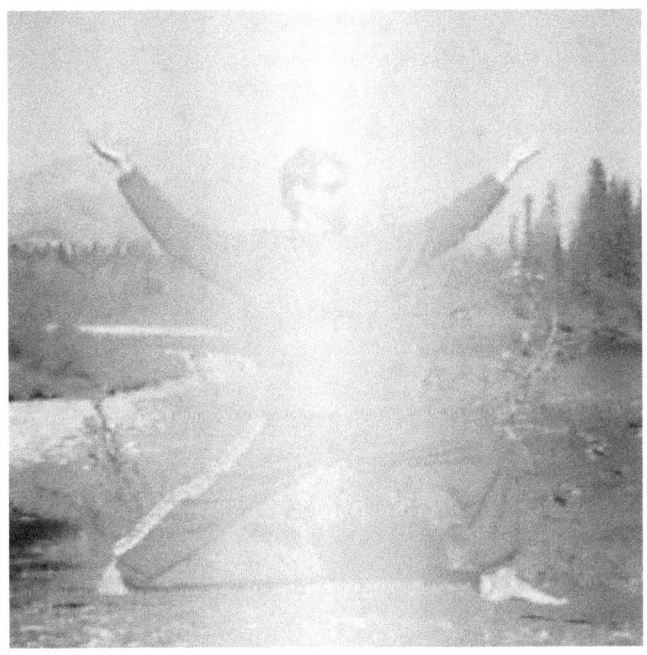

Figure 70: Shows an arm variation in Warrior 2 while
Conducting Heaven and Earth.

CHAPTER 22
INVERSIONS

I recommend always using a wall or some form of support with inversions so you do not fall backwards. It is commonly taught that it is safe to fall backwards the "right way", but many people still get minor injuries in their hands, neck and/or back when doing so. Please use a wall or another support until you are excellent at maintaining control in the inversions.

Details on Plough and Shoulder Stand

It is a good idea to raise your shoulders up to be a bit higher than the back of your head when in Plough and Shoulder Stand. This will reduce the strain on your neck. This can be achieved by folding in your mat or a towel.

Details on Heaven and Earth Exercises

In general, I do not recommend doing Heaven and Earth Exercises while inverted. Heaven and Earth Exercises can be done while inverted, by pulling Earth PE up into your feet and Heaven PE down to your head. This will challenge your control over PE. Never pull Earth PE into your head and down to your feet or Heaven PE into your feet towards your head. This can be compared to running electricity threw a computer backwards.

CHAPTER 23
FROM SEATED PART 2

The asanas from seated in this chapter have been separated from Chapter 15, because they are more commonly done near the end of an asana practice.

At the end of your practice, a seated Experiential Meditation and/or psychic energy exercise to facilitate balancing, harmonizing and integrating are very good to do. You will be in a great place for bringing completion to processes stared in your practice and empowering them. The Heaven and Earth Exercises are great for doing this. The Heaven PE will help fuel and refine changes, while the Earth PE empowers them.

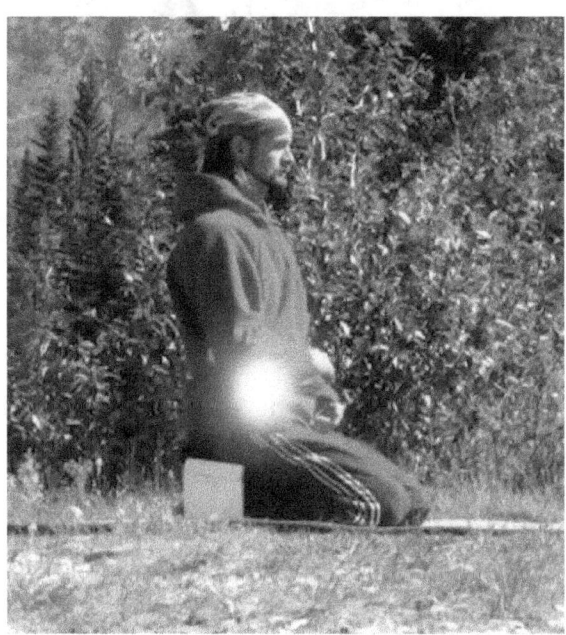

Figure 71: Charging the tan tien is a very common practice at the end of many practices involving PE. Doing so helps empower the new you.

Details on Hamstring Stretch

This is my own posture that is done like a standard hamstring stretch from gym class in high school, but your opposite hand presses into your bent leg helping to pull your spine out of your hips. Your arm can press harder than your lower back can handle, so be mindful. This can give great release to the lower back, especially when your practice also includes Pigeon or Half-Lotus on Your Back.

If the groin muscle is tight, this can help lengthen it as well.

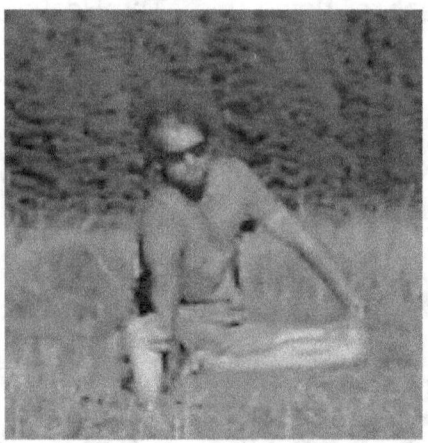

Figure 72: Shows a variation of Hamstring Stretch that helps pull the spine out of the hips by pressing on the opposite leg for leverage.

Details on Neck Stretches

By grabbing onto your ankles while kneeling or the side of a Kneeling Stool (figure 73), neck stretches can be made more intense. Be mindful of how hard you pull on your neck muscles, because these techniques give you way more potential power than your neck muscles can handle.

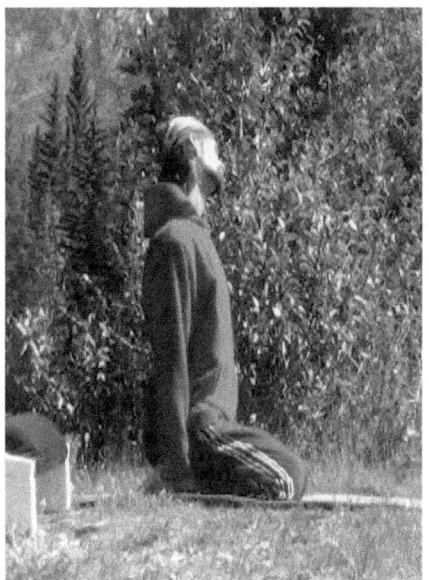 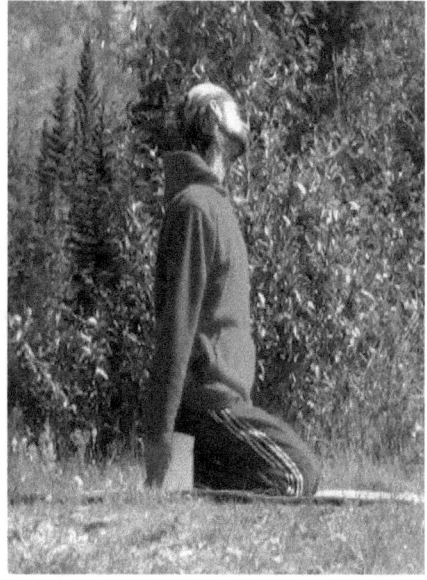

Figure 73: Show the use the ankle while kneeling (left) and the side of a Kneeling Stool (right) to intensify neck stretches.

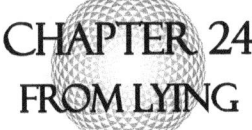

CHAPTER 24
FROM LYING

Details on Corpse

All the psychic energy exercises can be done in Corpse, in fact I encourage it, because it is easy to get really relaxed, which will improve your awareness and receptivity to PE. Holding your arms in place can get tiresome. I suggest using pillows and blankets to help hold your arms in place when necessary. I give a few example postures in the figures below. I give a few other examples in the Brain Enhancement Exercises in Appendix F .

Getting really relaxed is easier when meditating or doing psychic energy exercises. This makes it easy to fall a sleep afterward and during. For this reason, I recommend doing them while lying down (Corpse) before going to sleep for the night.

There is more to this than just falling asleep. It also helps prepare you for your higher self/soul to work with you more easily as you sleep. The abundance of healthy PE and the state of your psychic anatomy make this possible.

Upon waking up is also a great to do psychic energy exercise, because you are more in a meditative state naturally. Doing so will help bring completion and empower what happened during the night as well, giving you a great start to your day.

Corpse is a common asana to end an asana practice with. I recommend doing so with the intent of enhancing self awareness, harmony, balance and strength. You can also focus on Heaven and Earth Exercises to help cleanse and empower yourself. If you are a teacher, these are great things to include in a guided meditation at this time.

212

Most importantly! You must to remember this! You are not truly in Corpse unless you stop your heart and breath. Ohhhh yes. {Written with an Indian dialect ;) }[104]

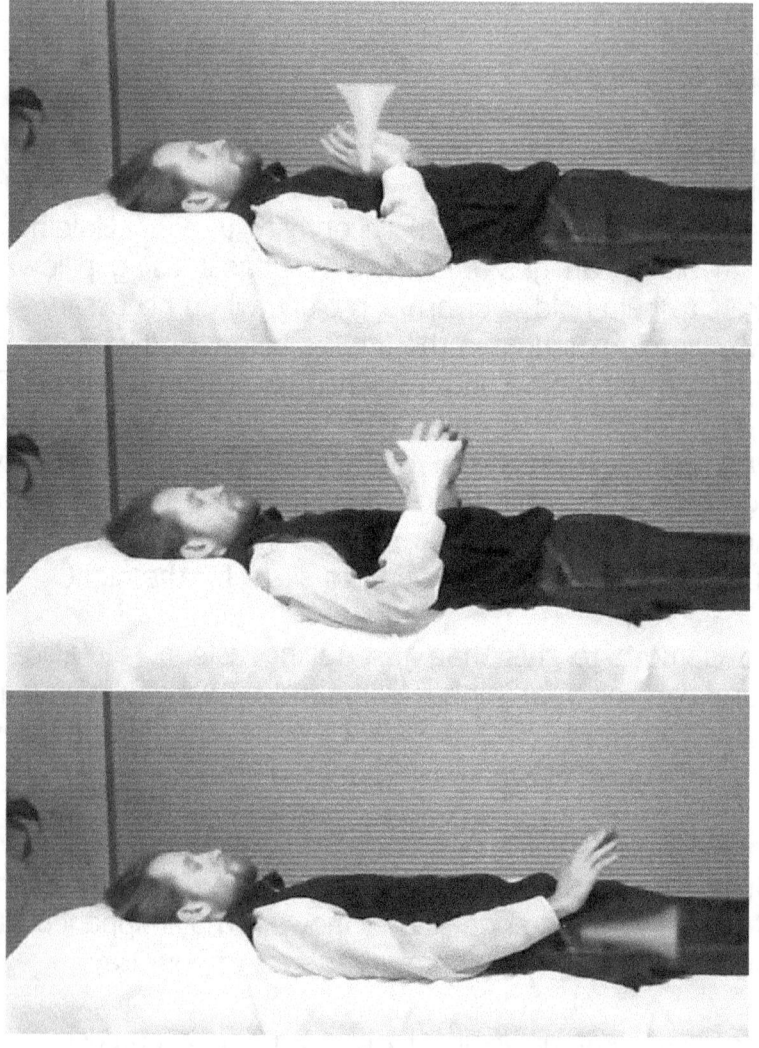

Figure 74: Working with chakras while in Corpse (lying down).

CHAPTER 25
PSYCHIC ANATOMY YOGA FLOWS

Psychic Anatomy Yoga flows are the same as regular yoga flows, except psychic energy exercises are incorporated between asanas or as a part of them. I have discussed a few flows below and have shared many in DVDs. Take your choice and make up your own.

Morning Routine

Step 1

Doing some of the psychic energy exercises from Part 1, Energy Healing and/or another practice of meditation/PE before getting out of bed is a great start (lying down or sitting up). This is a time when you are still well connected to your higher-self, because of the sleeping process. This gives you the advantage of being more receptive, aware and capable of working with PE.

During this time, abdominal breathing can be done to help get food in your digestive tract moving again. This works particularly well when vertical. It can result in gas being released and deep exhalations to occur as the digestive system starts to move food again as well as the movement of PE; the digestive system is closely connected to the digesting emotional and mental experiences in regards to PE.

If you get tired during this practice, let yourself fall back to sleep. It often results in waking up feeling awesome! If time does not permit this freedom, going to bed earlier might be a wise option. The healthier you are, the better life gets.

Step 2

You can start with this step is you wish.

Move to where you practice yoga and sit or stand with a vertical spine and focus on breathing with your whole body or just your abdomen. Drink some water as you do a General Alignment, Scanning and/or other sets of movements that has your hands moving between the top and bottom of your reach. Incorporate some gentle twists and leans as well. These movements will help awaken your digestive tract as the water moves threw it, as well as help awaken other parts of your body.

Do this for a few minutes or until you feel like your digestive tract has awakened and you have drunk enough water[105] then eat some fruit[106]. The fruit will awaken your blood with a balance of sugars and other nutrients that will also aid in the cleansing cycle[107]. In general, this is more true for organic fruits than those grown by industrial standards. It will also awaken your digestive system with enzymes and macrobiotics for your breakfast.

When eating your fruit, it is a good time to take cleansing herbs for your digestive system, because the fruit will travel quickly threw your digestive system, carrying the herbs with it to lower parts of your digestive system, such as your large intestine. This is very effective for killing parasites as the sugar stimulates them to absorb, taking in the anti-parasite herbs more easily. Aside from capsules, Super-Healthy Beverages discussed in Appendix D are great ways to take these herbs in.

If eating fruit is not yet a part of your lifestyle, I encourage you to make it so.

---

[105] See Appendix D for a discussion on drinking enough water during the day.
[106] See Appendix D for fruits that combine well.
[107] Discussed in Appendix D.

Step 3

After you have eaten some fruit, move onto your yoga practice. You may wish do your routine partially or completely before consuming fruit as well. You can also consume fruit every 10-20 minutes during your routine as discussed in Appendix D.

I recommend starting with simple and gentle exercises that have your spine, arms and legs moving to help awaken your body. Try tracing circles with your hips and/or parts of your spine and/or shoulders. This works great for awakening the torso, particularly the spine, which is a very important part.

Follow these movements with Threading the Needle, Side Stretches from Hands and Knees, Child's Pose, Down Dog and Lunge to fully awaken your torso, spine, hips and legs. These asanas do not need to be intense to be effective. In fact, in the morning, it is best to be gentle as circulation returns to these areas from a night of not moving. As you get warmed up, you can move onto more challenging asanas.

If you need to eat some fruit for energy before ingesting enough water, depending on how much fruit you have eaten and how it was combined, it may take 10-20 minutes for your stomach to be empty again[108]. As you develop your self-awareness, you'll be able to determine when your stomach is empty. It is best to drink enough water before eating the fruit, so the fruit's enzymes are in your stomach for breakfast.

---

[108] Discussed in Appendix D.

Step 4

Time for breakfast, which can be a Super-Healthy Beverage or Super-Healthy Salad. I have a collection of Super-Healthy Beverages and Salads that I share in Appendix D. In general, the drinks combine fruit, leafy vegetables and the super foods italian parsley, cilantro and sometimes garlic. These drinks digest quickly (~ 1.5-2 hours). Super-Healthy Salads combine a salad with super foods, powdered super foods and oils that give you a truly amazing start to your day.

Consume breakfast in a peaceful state and stay in a peaceful state for at least 10 minutes afterward to give your body a chance to get a good start on digesting your breakfast. It is always a good idea to sit peacefully after a meal. It can easily become a lengthy meditation, which is great timing for digestive purposes. This will give you optimal energy for your activities that follow.

Step 5

Have a great day :) !

Heat Series/Sun Salutations

In general, the psychic energy exercises in Part 1 are best done when your spine is vertical. The best time for doing this is when Standing.   Heat Series/Sun Salutations take you in and out of Standing several times. I recommend incorporating the General Routine split into pieces, so specific systems of your psychic anatomy (ex. aura, hara, core star, meridians, internal aura) are done each time you visit Standing.

Ending Your Practice

Near the end of your practice is a good time to start slowing down and focus on getting into a deeper meditative state. Less, slower and less challenging asanas are recommended. The goals is to find yourself into a place of stillness for Experiential Meditation and final psychic energy exercises. Remember that you can use your mind to do these exercises. The movements and postures are only for amplification.

Ending Your Day

It is important to clear, balance and center yourself before going to bed. This will give you a better night's sleep. An intense physical practice can help as well, relieving stress and tiring the body. Doing the psychic energy exercises from Part 1 intensely can as well, but sometimes it will electrify your senses, making it harder to sleep. In time you will learn to sleep in these states more easily and sometimes you will stay just above falling asleep, sometimes willingly, doing these exercises intuitively and/or other practices of PE (ex. energy healing[109]) for several hours.

These can be awesome experiences! Blessings in disguise. When having these experiences, you are in the deepest meditative state you can be in before falling asleep, which empowers your abilities. When I have these experiences, I often feel euphoric, balanced and strong the next day.

Having a calming and centering night routine, such as reading something calming and educational will help you fall asleep and sleep well. Do not participate in anything that could be an unhealthy influence, such as watching certain TV shows/movies, playing certain games or eating unhealthily (the last thing you

---

[109] Energy Healing discussed in *Psychic Anatomy Treatments*.

eat should be very nutritious and support sleep actives[110]). Only expose yourself to health influences, especially before just before going to sleep or entering a post meditative state before sleeping. Studying is a great example, assuming you are not too tired. If you are tired, meditating for the evening could be your best choice.

Having a consistent sleeping schedule helps a lot as well. Your bodies work on rhythms and if sleeping and eating rhythms are consistent, it gets easier for your body to function, improving mind-body-spirit health and performance in many ways.

You should wake up feeling rejuvenated every morning. If not, go to bed earlier and/or change your evening habits. Quality sleep can make a significant difference to your health and performance, especially over longer periods of time!

Making sure you are sufficiently fed and watered will also improve sleep quality. Hunger can cause discomfort that can awaken you, interrupting your sleep. If you need to eat within the last 3-4 hours of your day, make it just vegetables, because they digest in 2 hours. If you need something denser, yogurt and other liquify options (ex protein shakes) are good choices. In general, these options are easy to move out of the stomach.

Foods that do not move out of the stomach easily can get over digested and toxic. They are also harder to move threw the intestines, causing discomfort. Sleeping while sitting up or on your right side can help get food out of your stomach while sleeping.

Over watering can cause you to get up to urinate during the night, but it is worth it if your body needs water. Just get up slowly, walk slowly and try to stay just above a state of sleep, making it easier to return to sleep. Your body detoxifies as you sleep, so adequate water is necessary. Obviously it is best to

---

[110] Discussed in *Becoming Super Human.*

have enough water during the day, making less water needed at night.

Detoxification supplements, such as the Super Healthy Beverages discussed in Appendix D can be beneficial. This will most likely have you getting up at least once to urinate, but it will also help you detox, which is really important for some people.

At night your body also focuses on regenerating its reserves of important molecules as well as cell division. Taking a multivitamin or half of one can help support these processes without needing to ingest food. See my book *Becoming Super Human* for more information of supplementing at night.

CHAPTER 26
FINAL COMMENTS

For some people, this book has presented a lot of new information. This type of information can result in a lot changes to occur in your life as you become aware of these parts of yourself and reality. Be patient and mindful with yourself as these changes occur, making time for reflection, rejuvenation and integration. This is an amazing and sometimes challenging process that continues to develop in its magnificence and potential as you do.

You are worth every bit of effort you put into yourself. May the information in this and my other books fuel your efforts with motivation and guidance to make living to your fullest potential as an unique individual as easy and effective as possible.

Namaste.

- - - APPENDICES - - -

APPENDIX A
GROUP PRACTICE

Practicing in a group is highly recommended, because everyone in the group contributes to the collective field of PE, increasing the abundance, diversity, balance, harmony and power of healthy PE for everyone to work with. Even if it is just for one night a week or month, group practice of Psychic Anatomy Yoga or just the psychic energy exercises of Part 1[111], is well worth the effort for everyone involved. It will make it easier to overcome barriers in your private practice that can be integrated with and refined more precisely later on in your private practice if necessary.

A person's home is usually where group practices occur. This has some advantages to the group and of course the person's home. A person's home usually has less activity than a public space, which allows for the environment's psychic anatomy to develop more with less maintenance. The psychic anatomy of the house/room develops to be in harmony with the group, making it easier for the group to work together.

Choose a home that is already kept clean, organized and doesn't have much activity. If you know a person who is very engaged in Psychic Anatomy Yoga, a similar practice and/or is introverted and observant, they make excellent keepers of these spaces, because they usually continue to work with it consciously and unconsciously between group practices. These people will have a great advantage by living within this space, because of the increased power and harmony pf PE.

Some people will not like having their environment disturbed. If you have an excellent home to share I encourage you to learn to work with groups and share your environment with the intent

---

[111] See *The Psychic Anatomy Exercises* for more exercises like these.

of serving our collective evolution. Rarely will the group lessen the quality of your environment, but in the long run, they will more than likely help improve it. The only challenge will be clearing released unhealthy PE and harmonizing with the elevated power of PE. It is good practice to include some environmental exercises at the end of group practice for these reasons.

As your group gets better at Psychic Anatomy Yoga, it may feel guided to do environmental work from a distance or go to areas in person. Having group practice in public spaces will enhance the health and performance of its psychic anatomy, which will benefits everyone who experiences it. The only disadvantage is to beginner groups, because the psychic anatomy of the environment will not be as compatible to their development, because of all the traffic public spaces experience. With a few experienced people, this can easily be over come.

MedMob.org is a group that organizes public meditations in public spaces with the intent of enhancing our collective evolution. They make use of the Maharishi Effect[112], which is the phenomenon of a group empowering PE in an environment to create positive change. They are a good group to work with.

FYI: Environmental exercises are discussed in more detail within *The Psychic Anatomy Exercises.*

When it comes to choosing a leader, I recommend trying to get everyone involved in leading the group periodically. Some will have more skills than others for leading the group and they will naturally take more of a leadership role. This is fine, but these people must be mindful of the benefits of helping others learn to lead.

Once everyone is connected in a meditative state, the PE could resonant with different people better, making them opportune people to guide the practice further. I have done many

---

[112] Search Maharishi Effect online.

practices like this and highly recommend this approach. Assuming ego does not resist people contributing or encourage them to over contribute.

Remember the importance of preparation work. In group situations the collective consciousness makes it easier for those of less health and performance to contribute without causing harm; assuming the group's collective consciousness is predominantly healthy. This is important to know when some people are transitioning into a healthier state and may be detoxifying.

There is less connection between group members in the beginning of the practice and the first part is usually individual based, which gives time and freedom for people to get ready to optimize themselves to be a healthy contribution to the group's collective consciousness. Still it is best to do some preparation work before joining the group environment.

I recommend reading *Psychic Anatomy Treatments* for more information on working with groups from an energy healing perspective.

APPENDIX B
GROUP EXERCISES

These group exercises are intended as warm-up exercises. They will help unify the group as well as help develop awareness and control of PE.

Building and Manipulating a Sphere of Psychic Energies

The most common game is taught in Chapter 2 as a warm up. It uses Pulsating or Pulsate Breathing to build a sphere of PE between your hands. Often people notice a tingling, pressure, temperature change or another sensation as their psychic anatomy is stimulated and awakened at their hands.

With practice, a group can combine their spheres together and/or pass spheres around. They can also push upon spheres creating gentle waves within them. This needs to be done gently, because pushing too fast will have you push right threw it.

Building a Circuit

Eeman, in 1947, found that the electric potential of the human body could be used to promote relaxation or tension by placing the left or right hands on the head or hips. Specifically, placing the left hand on the head and right hand on the hips promoted relaxation and the opposite promoted tension; this is reverse for left handed people[113]. This works for placing hands anywhere on the body as well. As long as the left is higher, relaxation will be promoted.

---

[113] Discussed in more details within *The Psychic Energy Reality* (Appendix H) and *The Interface Between Psychic Energies and the Physical Body.*

This worked for individuals and groups. Have a group place their left hand on their neighbors shoulder and their right hand their opposite neighbor's hip, thigh or knee. Left handed people will place their hands in reverse. Get the group to focus on the same intentions, such as entering a meditative state and the PE will circulate around the circle promoting this state.

You can try a variation of this exercise by hovering hands just above their neighbors shoulder/hips. This will require more of their psychic anatomy to create the connection.

Remember to do a preparation exercise before this to make sure the circulating PE are predominantly healthy.

Winds of Psychic Energies

PE don't need to be channeled threw you for you to control them. If you focus on winds of PE swirling around you, someone else or in an environment, you can make it happen. This is a more advanced technique, but some people can do it easily. Doing it as a group makes it easier and more powerful. Be mindful of your intentions. The goal is to enhance health and performance with respect to evolution, not to be noticed.

Incorporating Essential Oils

Doing the exercises above with essential oils in the air or on your hands can alter/enhance the PE being worked with. This is a fun way to develop your awareness, because they can greatly change the types of PE present. Using Essential Oils in this way can be incorporated into Psychic Anatomy Yoga as well.

Incorporating Gemstones

Incorporating gemstones has a similar effect as essential oils. The main difference is that they need to be charged with PE. This needs to be done carefully with some people present, because they can be very powerful amplifiers, too powerful for some people, influencing them into a state of Qi-Gong Psychosis (discussed in Appendix C). Remember that balanced and harmonized power is much easier to handle. Make it a high priority.

When it comes to groups working with gemstones, geometry of their placement is important. There can be one gemstones or grid of them in the center of the group and/or a grid surrounding the group. Other good places are on walls, corners of rooms, over door ways and windows and/or on clean-clear table in the practice space. The goal is to have them in the open so PE can easily access them. This will make it easier for them to resonant with PE naturally.

With balance, harmony and purity as a priority, the group can focus on cultivating specific types of PE (ex. those that can help the group live to their fullest potential) and once they have been cultivated, the gemstones will resonant with them naturally, especially when placed symmetrically with the group. They can also be focused into them with the intention to do so. This is a more powerful way to do so, but not always as pure.

The reason for this potential purity decrease is that we are imperfect. When we focus PE into gemstones, there is more of a connection made with them, which makes it possible for the PE of our imperfections to be amplified by them. When the connection is less direct, higher aspects of our consciousness to refine the resonance in the gemstones to be more optimal.

Gemstones are truly amazing tools to work with. As you learn to work with them and PE in general, you will become more masterful and the potential benefits of working with them will improve as well.

I recommend students bring their own gemstones to be apart of this experience. It will make it easier to maintain the presence of these PE within them once leaving the group practice. I recommend that they focus on the intention of their personal gemstone only picking up on the PE that will help them and all they interact with to live to their fullest potential.

When it comes to choosing gemstones, I recommend clear quartz, because it is the most versatile. There are many books on the properties of gemstones. The best way to use them is with developed awareness of PE and self. Every stone can be complimentary at the right time and for the right amount of time. When it comes to group work, try just using clear quartz and maybe rose quartz and amethyst as well. This will keep things simple that you can expand upon in the future.

A good way to use gemstones, such as clear quartz, is to wear them around your neck as a pendulum. Wearing them will amplify the PE in your psychic anatomy. This is especially beneficial for helping to maintain the presence of PE cultivated during your group or personal practice after your practice. It is not always best to wear them during the practice though, because of potential unhealthy PE being released, getting overwhelmed by the amplification and avoiding potential dependence upon them.

Like your psychic anatomy, gemstones can get congested with unhealthy PE, especially if you are detoxifying unhealthy PE while wearing them or have them near by. The best way to keep them clear is to keep yourself clear. If you are detoxifying, give some attention to clearing your gemstones and of course yourself. Flush them with the healthy PE you are cultivating and when this is not working, using salt, salt water, running water and sunlight are effective ways to clear gemstones as well. Just place them in the salt, salt water, running water or sunlight with the intent clearing them[114].

---

[114] Amethyst is bleached by direct sunlight. Do not expose to direct sunlight.

APPENDIX C
BECOMING A TEACHER

Being a dedicated teacher to a group is very different compared to leading a group as discussed in Appendix A. As a teacher, you could be teaching people with no conscious experience with PE[115], people who are very unhealthy and groups that are difficult to harmonize. This requires you to be educated and powerful with PE. It also requires you to be in a healthy state of health and performance.

Teaching is very similar to energy healing-empowerment. There is a transfer of PE between teacher and students. If the teacher is unhealthy, it is likely that they will transfer unhealthy PE as they teach. I talk about this in more detail within *Psychic Anatomy Treatments* (energy healing-empowerment treatments is an even more sensitive situation in this regards).

Your knowledge of Psychic Anatomy Yoga is your foundation. Upon it, awareness and control of PE are your next most valuable skills. Self-awareness of how you respond to Psychic Anatomy Yoga techniques and PE is in general is much easier than becoming aware of how your students respond in these ways. Some people have this ability naturally, others develop it really quickly and for others it takes longer.

Some people's awareness works in a way that makes them susceptible to taking on other people's PE. These people need to learn to control their receptiveness before they can be effective teachers. This involves controlling how open their heart chakra is to certain types of PE, as well as controlling how much attention they give to experiences. You need to be able to let go immediately. A valuable skill for life in general.

---

[115] Everybody experiences PE unconsciously.

Teachers need to be aware of their student's level of development and the experiences they are having as the group practices for optimal results. If a student's foundation is not ready for the power a group cultivates, it can be very discomforting. This is especially true when students are new to these experiences. Making quality a much higher priority than power can help insure a pleasant experiences for everyone.

Making time to help comfort a student when they look distressed is recommended. It is also a good idea to talk with them after class as well. Often they will just need their experience(s) validated and/or explained to them to bring them comfort. Your knowledge of the information presented in this book, as well as my others, will prepare you with a great foundation of knowledge to draw upon in these situations.

There is great power in numbers when it comes to all practices of PE. A teacher's awareness and power to control the PE in the group's collective consciousness can help avoid discomforting experiences for all group members. The best way to do this is to work with the field of collective consciousness directly, helping to maintain its balance, harmony and purity.

As you become aware of the quality of the collective field, you are tuned into it and can change it by focusing your attention on improving it both collectively and locally. An example of locally would be the space around a person(s) rather than the entire group.

These techniques are easier for some to develop than others. The environmental exercises discussed in Chapter 16 of *Psychic Anatomy Treatments* are great exercises for developing these skills.

Sometimes students will need your direct support, requiring you to move into their space, using your hands (ex. General Techniques) to focus and move PE. Knowledge and experience with the information in *Psychic Anatomy Treatments* and other Energy Healing modalities can help a lot in these situations. Often these experiences will be brief, helping them finish off the healing and/or awakening experience they are having. Leaving them in a balanced and harmonized state.

Intense healing and awakening experiences can leave a person feeling uncomfortable/overwhelmed. This is different to Qi-Gong Psychosis, which is discussed below. Familiarity with healing and awakening experiences makes you more capable to comfort and reassure a person who is unfamiliar with them, as well as prepare them in advance to have them. Often intuition will guide you in these moments for what to and not to say/do.

Be mindful that working with people directly, and as groups to a degree, can be a sexually arousing experience. Beautiful energies are interacting, sometimes for the purpose of healing, which makes connecting an unwise thing to do[116]. Never act on these sensations without consent. It is very possible that the other person, especially if they are not as aware of PE as you are and/or having a healing experience, is not experiencing the same thing.

While helping an individual, it is best to stay connected to the group as a whole. Changes in them could catalyze changes in others. We are all connected.

You need to be mindful of how much your students can handle. Overloading them physically is not a big deal. Mentally is not a big deal for most people either, but overloading their psychic anatomy is unfamiliar to most, which can make it a big deal.

Overloading a person's psychic anatomy is recognized in psychology as "Qi-Gong Psychosis[117]". Qi-Gong Psychosis

---

[116] When people are healing, unhealthy PE can be released, which you can absorb if trying to connect.

[117] DSM, 1994, *Diagnostic and Statistical Manual of Mental Disorders, fourth ed*, Washington, D.C.: The American Psychiatric Association, p. 847.

describes an scattered-spinning state of mind that is the result of being overwhelmed by too much psychic energy and/or changes to your psychic anatomy[118]. This is rare, but more common when over practicing or in groups that can build strong fields of PE, neglecting balance, harmony and purity. Quality before quantity is a good general rule to follow.

A teacher can make it much easier on themselves in this way by making it a priority to bring the group individuals into a state of optimal balance, harmony and purity before beginning the practice.

Following this process, you can guide the group into state of group coherence. I recommend the HeartMath approach of focusing healthy PE on the physical heart, such as the PE associated with the emotions of love, compassion, patience and other virtues. This has been observed by HeartMath to influence bioelectric coherence in the entire body and brain. Once this is accomplished, group coherence happens naturally more easily as well, which can be noticed as everyone breathing in coherence, the feel of the collective consciousness and sometimes synchronicity.

If the group needs some helping reaching a state of group coherence, getting them to focus on the same intentions and/or having them chant or tone together can help. Other group exercises are discussed in Appendix B.

Another approach that can make it easier on the teacher to create and maintain balance, harmony and purity, is teaching the students to make it a priority. I recommend teaching students to use the Fundamental Affirmations (Chapter 2) as well as the self-help techniques discussed in *Inner and Outer Success* and other resources to help maintain and enhance these states of being within themselves.

---

[118] Healing and empowerment cause psychic anatomy to restructure.

These affirmations and techniques can also help after group practice, which is an even more important time to use them for some people. Group practice tends to leave student's psychic anatomy in expanded states as their psychic anatomy changes to resonant (integrate/embody) with a higher quality and quantity of PE. This can make them more sensitive to external influences that could imbalance, disharmony and pollute them. Especially the techniques in *Inner and Outer Success* can help avoid this.

The lack of support of the group's collective consciousness also makes them more sensitive as they are now more independently maintaining the presence of the higher quality and quantity of PE within themselves as they try to integrate with them. For these reasons, I recommend making time after class for students to meditate in stillness as they integrate and ground. I also recommend they remain this state and minimize external influences for as long as they feel necessary once leaving.

Your practice/teaching space should be a sacred space. Some spaces, like those in nature, already hold an abundance of healthy PE and are complimentary to cultivating healthy PE. Some places need to be periodically cleared and charged with healthy PE. Either way, your practice/teaching space should be charged with healthy PE before and/or during the warm up routine (warm-up routine: creating individual balance, harmony and purity and then group coherence) and maintained during.

At the certification workshops, you will spend time with me and other people practiced Psychic Anatomy Yoga and related arts. A truly wonderful experience that can greatly enhance your personal development with the potential of all the extraordinary people and the PE they embody. There will be several opportunities dedicated to optimizing this.

Teacher Certification

Becoming a teacher of Psychic Anatomy Yoga is an easy process for some, but not for all. The abilities for helping people one-on-one and collectively to develop their knowledge and skills takes many skills on your end; discussed above. As you develop these skills, there are 4 Levels of certification to go through.

Level 1

For Level 1 certification, you are required to show that you have memorized the teachings of Psychic Anatomy Yoga and can teach them in a workshop and class setting. You will need to submit an essay explaining your approach to teaching a beginners group and how you would progress from day one, leading them towards becoming experts. This essay will help you organize your thoughts, consider situations that you may over look otherwise and help you manifest becoming a teacher[119].

When you are at the certification workshop, you will need to teach a class of peers and volunteers, answer questions and contribute to discussions.

With Level 1 certification, you are approved to teach classes of up to 5 people.

Level 2

Level 2 requires you to display your abilities to work with environments, fields of collective consciousness and individuals in the ways discussed above. These are very important skills.

---

[119] Manifestation teachings often use essays, dream boards and other physical expressions to empower the PE associated with what is trying to be manifested.

Level 2 certification approves you to teach up to 15 people.

Level 2 teachers can team up with other approved teachers to teach groups equal to the summation of all teachers involved. For example, two Level 2 teachers can teach 30 people. I recommend having one lead the group and the others focusing on supporting individuals, the environment and the group's collective consciousness. It awesome to teach this way!

Level 3

You will need to submit videos of yourself teaching 3 classes, one workshop and give an introduction to yourself on them. Please make sure your audio recording is done well.

At the certification workshop you will display your Level 2 abilities again. This routine will display your abilities, health and performance (ex. activations of upper soul gates).

There is no maximum number to the group sizes of Level 3 teachers. It will be up to you to determine how many people you can work with optimally.

Remember, the more students you have the more difficult it can be to maintain an optimal environment and sufficient attention to individual students. This is even more true when group coherence is hard to achieve and maintain and/or many group members are releasing unhealthy PE. Teaming up with other teachers can greatly help, as can maintaining a core group of experienced people in your classes and introducing new people mindfully.

Level 4

Level 4 certification allows you to certify other teachers. This is something I decide after getting to know you.

Psychic Anatomy Exercises/Treatment Certification

Once you are certified to teach Psychic Anatomy Yoga, you are closer to being certified for Psychic Anatomy Exercises/Treatments as well. Certification in these practices will play an important role in receiving Level 4 certification. See my books *The Psychic Anatomy Exercises* and *Psychic Anatomy Treatments* for details.

Psychic Anatomy Exercises Teacher Certification

Teaching Psychic Anatomy Exercises is different compared to Psychic Anatomy Yoga, because there are no asanas. This is both an advantage and disadvantage. Without asanas the student spends more time in stillness and can get very ungrounded. Their teacher needs to teach them about and help them with these experiences and how to return to a balance, harmonized and a grounded state afterward. To be certified to teach Psychic Anatomy Exercises on their own, you need to show the same skills as for Psychic Anatomy Yoga, but be more masterful with them.

APPENDIX D
HEALTHY DIET HINTS

There is lots of information out there on healthy diet hints. These subjects are a major focus on mine that I have been studying since 2001. Below is a summary of some of the more important topics. In my book *Becoming Super Human* I review more advanced topics.

Healthy-Inexpensive Ingredients

Sprouts

Sprouts are extremely healthy and inexpensive. I recommend making them a staple in your diet. A salad composed of primarily sprouts and some other vegetables is a great meal for freshness, energy and feeling awesome afterward.

Essentially sprouts are are baby plants, which are high in protein, vitamins, minerals, enzymes[120] and other nutrients. The way they are made is by soaking a seed, nut or bean that sprouts (ex. lentil, mung bean, sun flower seed; see internet for details) for about 10 hours, draining them and then rinsing them every 6-10 hours or when they look dry; there is no risk of over rinsing them. Keep doing this until their roots are a bit longer than the body or until they are sprouted just the way you like them.

The examples above can be eaten raw (lentils are fantastic!), but others require at least 3 minutes of steaming/boiling to make them more edible (see internet for details). Once sprouted they will keep in excellent shape for about 5 days in the fridge and even longer if they are rinsed every 5 days.

---

[120] Enzymes are very important nutrients that are easily destroyed when food is heated over 115° F. Discussed again below with raw food.

Sprouts can be added to most salads and grain dishes. They can also be blended with some oil, water and/or butter to make an awesome hummus!!! I recommend adding salt, lemon juice and sometimes garlic for taste and health benefits. Many herbs will combine well into these hummuses (ex. italian parsley and cilantro). Remember that less is often better, especially when you are learning how to make them.

Raw Foods

The idea with raw foods is that nothing is cooked that doesn't have to be cooked in order to maximize nutrients sensitive to heat, specifically enzymes. Enzyme help breakdown food and other substances (ex. farm chemicals, germs and other toxins). When you get them from your food, your body has to work less at making its own, which gives you more energy to devote to using the abundance of nutrients you have taken in.

Often people will detoxify when they are moving into a raw food diet. The extra energy and increase in nutrients causes your body to start detoxifying in the background of it regular activities. This can be an overwhelming experience for people with lots of toxicity. Drinking more water can help a lot. Once your body has purged enough toxins, raw foods will not stimulate detoxification and cleanses are needed for deeper cleansing; discussed below.

I recommend slowly moving into a raw food diet by cooking vegetables/foods less and less until you are on a pure raw food diet. Please note that some foods need to be cooked, such as legumes (beans), squash and most grains. Find a raw food book for details or search the internet.

In general, if you cook your food (veggies, grains, legumes, proteins) at less than 115°F you'll maintain the bulk of their enzymes, but not necessarily their life force. Slow cooker books might have more information on this than raw food ones. Please note that you can cook food slowly on a stove top and in a toaster/regular oven as well. A slow cooker is not always necessary. Even if we are above 115 C, the lower the temperature is the more nutrition that will be maintained.

Dried Beans

Dried beans taste much, much better than tinned beans and they are healthier[121] and less expensive[122] as well. Simply cover some dried beans with water and leave them for 6-8 hours (up to 24 hours is fine, can put in fridge to extend tend this time a little) and then cook them as slow as possible until tender. When the beans are evenly wet on the inside, they are done. If they are a little dry or hard they will likely give you gas.

Soaked Nuts and Seeds

Soaking nuts and seeds for 6-10 hours destroys the majority of the enzyme inhibitors, making them easier to digest. You can eat them as is, with other meals or blend them into a smoothie (smoothies discussed below).

Super-Healthy Beverages

These super healthy beverages can be consumed as an appetizer, when your diet is not as healthy as it could be or as a medicine when feeling run down. They can be as simple as putting cilantro and italian parsley into a blender with some water and adding fresh lemon and/or lime juice afterward and

---

[121] Tinned foods tend to leach tin, other metals and/or teflon into the food they contain. This is why many people do not buy dented cans! Tinned food is also less fresh, decreasing nutritional and life force value.

[122] Over time the approximate 50% saving can really add up, especially if beans are consumed regularly.

as complex as adding other fresh herbs, seeds and nuts. Cilantro and italian parsley are the two main herbs in my opinion, because they are readily available, inexpensive and packed with general health enhancing benefits. I'll talk a little about these and other ingredients below as I describe how to make these beverages.

Lettuce and Fruit Smoothies

These are probably the most amazing breakfast smoothies ever. Once pureed, the nutrients from these fresh foods will enter the body quickly, giving you a rush of nutrients and energy. Add chopped up apple, pear and/or other fruits[123] to a blender then then add lettuce, fresh cilantro, italian parsley and/or other herbs and puree with water. Its that simple and all it takes is the rinsing of the blender, cutting board and knife to clean up afterward.

Cilantro and italian parsley Drinks (Super Healthy and Detoxifying)

These are essentially the same drinks as above, but fruit is not an ingredient and lettuces do no have to be either. Cilantro and italian parsley are two of the most incredible herbs that you can get fresh at your grocery store for about a dollar each. These super herbs have been found to have a wide variety of health benefits to your entire body. Cilantro has a unique ability to help release heavy metals from your body, which is very important, because they are very toxic.

The metal releasing ability of cilantro is very strong, but it needs to be complimented with another herb that is high in chlorophyll, such as italian parsley, to help get them out of the

---

[123] Not all fruits combine well together when it comes to digestion. Food combining discussed below.

body[124]. If you drink a lot of cilantro juice without the extra chlorophyll, the metals can be reabsorbed by your body before being urinated out, which can result in you feeling sick; this is called reintoxication. Likewise, if you drink too much of any these Super-Healthy Beverage, your body can be overwhelmed, giving you a similar feeling. This is a similar concept to detoxification triggered by raw food diets; discussed above.

Another great herb to help get heavy metals out of our body is garlic. When it comes to detoxifying heavy metals it helps oxidate them, making it easier for the body to urinate them out. Both the Cilantro-italian parsley and Cilantro-italian parsley-Garlic drinks can be complimented with fresh lemon and/or lime juice, which are also super foods.

Note, these Cilantro-italian parsley drinks would not even be close to the same power or fresh taste if dried cilantro and italian parsley were used. Fresh is always better!

Cilantro-italian parsley Drink:
    Approx. ½ cup of loose cilantro leaves (some stem is OK)
    Approx. ½ cup of loose italian parsley[125] leaves (some stem is OK)
    Cover with water
    Liquefy in blender
    Add as much lemon as we want
    Consume*

Cilantro-italian parsley-Garlic Drink:
    Approx. ½ cup of loose cilantro leaves

---

[124] Both cilantro and italian parsley are high in chlorophyll, but cilantro is not high enough.
[125] I recommend a soft leave italian parsley, such as Italian italian parsley.

> Approx. ½ cup of loose italian parsley leaves (some stem is OK)
> Clove of chopped up garlic
> Cover with water
> Liquefy in blender
> Add as much lemon as we want
> Consume*
>
> ♦   *Consuming these drinks once a day is fine, but listen to your body. If it wants more or less listen. Sometimes these drinks will trigger rapid detoxification, depending on how toxic you are. If rapid detox happens, drink more water with lemon to help your body neutralize the toxins and release them.*
>
> *Note: Other ingredients can be added to these drinks. I'll discuss doing so below*

Any vegetable can be added to these smoothies, such as grated carrot, chopped celery and more. The catch is that making them taste good is more challenging. One of the advantages of pureeing veggies is that you'll get more nutrients from them, because they will be absorbed faster, avoiding nutrient breakdown from stomach acids.

Once you get good at making these drinks, they can be an incredible rush. My friends and I have consumed the cilantro-italian parsley drinks when feeling exhausted or slightly ill and it has greatly improved our sense of well-being. These are truly amazing drinks! Be patient and start with the guidelines I have given, adding other ingredients slowly.

Adding Seeds and Nuts

It is becoming common knowledge that essential fatty acids, such Omega 3, 6, 9, Epsychic anatomy and DHA are very important for maintaining physical health and performance. These nutrients are very sensitive to heat, causing them to be rare in many people's diets that do not contain a large amount of raw or semi-raw[126] foods.

Fatty acids help the cells in your body maintain their membranes, which improves their ability to communicate with each other and protect themselves from viruses, bacteria, fungus and toxins. Hemp hearts, flax seeds and chia seeds are both very high in essential fatty acids. Most seeds and nuts are high in them as well.

Making drinks and adding these foods to meals will help increase your essential fatty acid intake and improve general health and performance. I often will combine hemp hearts in with italian parsley and cilantro drinks, because hemp hearts are a very soft seed and when liquefied make a very nice texture and taste. Lemon and/or lime juice can also be added as well. Flax seeds are not the same. They need a coffee grinder to make them into a flour before adding them to a drink or to be soaked for 6-36 hours and then pureed in a blender.

I prefer the pre-soaking of flax/chia seeds[127] and then puree them with some soaked nuts, soaked seeds, coco, carob, maca root powder and/or sweetener to make the most amazing milk shake!! Since flax seeds are much less expensive than hemp seeds and chia seeds, I often choose flax seeds. Although hemp hearts have a great taste and texture.

---

[126] Semi-Raw implies coked below 115C (slow-cooked)
[127] Soaking also activate the sprouting process, making them easier to digest and more nutritious.

Some companies are trying to sell pre-ground hemp/flax seeds and hemp/flax seed oil[128]. The problem with these products is they do not contain any natural antioxidants, which means when oxidation happens after opening them, the damage doesn't stop and the oil starts to rot/decay quickly. This is why they recommend to keep these products in the freezer and consume them quickly. It makes more sense for health, nutrition and cost to buy flax seeds, chia seeds and hemp hearts whole and use them as I have suggested.

Note: You can buy EPA/DHA essential fatty acid gel capsule supplements as well. These fatty acids can really enhance and maintain brain health and performance[129]. Some fish have these specific essential fatty acids in large amounts, but when they are cooked lots of these oils will break down. Supplements are the best way to get lots of them.

Super-Healthy Salads

Any salad is a good meal, but they are not always filling. Adding the super foods avocado, soaked nuts and seeds, ground flax, spirulina, chlorella and/or other super foods can really step up a salad. I have one almost every morning. Of course, italian parsley, cilantro and garlic are usually added as well.

My personal favorite combination is ground flax, spirulina, sea salt[130] and extra virgin olive oil on top of a salad that I mix together. Amazing! Other ingredients work with this combination as well, although I do need to be mindful of not making it too oily when adding avocado.

---

[128] In gel capsules are OK, but are very expensive in comparison.

[129] These fish oils do not naturally contain natural antioxidants and decay quickly. This is why gel capsules are recommended over bottles of oil. If we are consuming them quickly, bottles of oil are more economical.

[130] Sea salt can really bring out taste in a salad.

There are many powdered super foods that can be added to a salad. We just need to experiment a little to find a taste and texture that we can work with. Remember to make food a priority as fuel, not entertainment. We can have both, but we might need to persevere until we find combinations that work. It gets easier after awhile.

Important Diet Concepts

Sufficient **Water** intake is very important to bodily function, especially when detoxifying and/or working hard. Drinking water with meals is in general and bad idea, because it dilutes digestive fluids, which can make you feel tired after eating. Sometimes it is a good idea to drink a small amount of water with a meal. Such a time is when your body is low on water and your meal feels dry in your stomach. It can also be a good idea to periodically sip on water between meals to help flush/absorb nutrients out of the stomach, protecting them from being over digested.

In general, the morning and before meals is the best time to consume large amounts of water, because your stomach is empty. How much water you need depends on many things. In general, if your urine is coming out clear twice in a row, then you are getting more than enough water. Anywhere between 1-3 liters/day can be expected.

Food combining is the science of combining foods for optimal digestion. It is as simple as finding the chart on the internet and printing it out so you can reference it when planning meals. The most important is to avoid combining dense proteins and carbohydrates. When combined, digestion does not occur as well, resulting in more energy being needed for digestion, longer digestion times, lower quality of digestion and more. Other general rules are shown in the chart below. See

256

Becoming Super Human for more information on food combining and other diet hints.

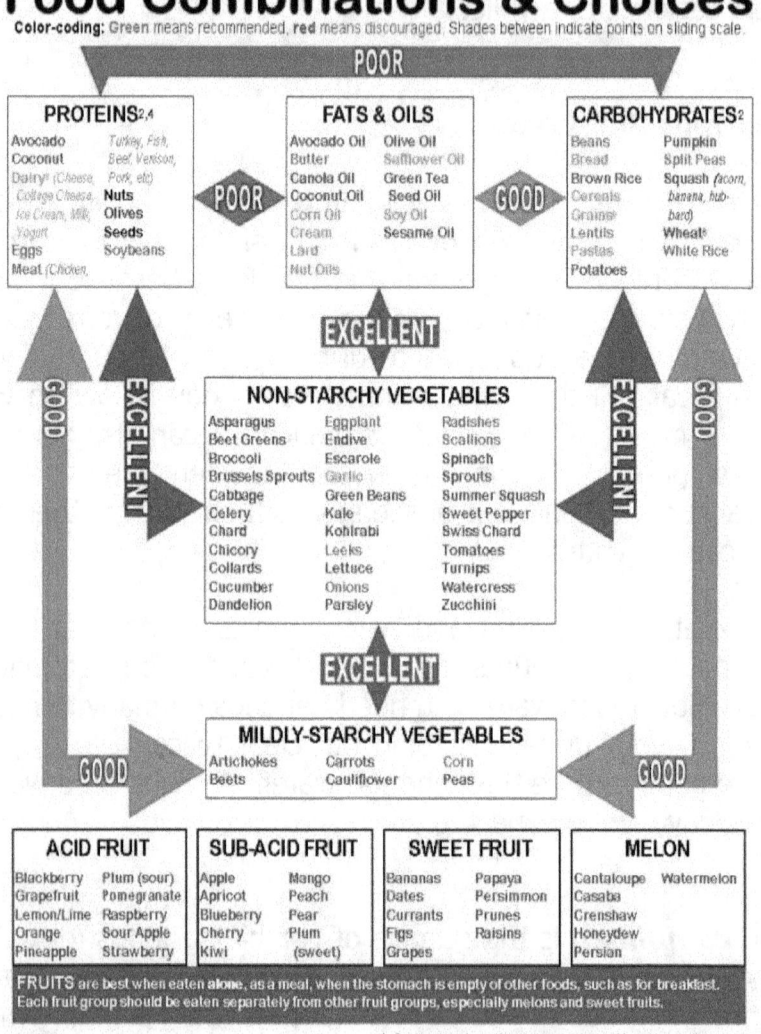

Food Combinations & Choices

Color-coding: Green means recommended, red means discouraged. Shades between indicate points on sliding scale.

POOR

PROTEINS[2,4]

Avocado	*Turkey, Fish,*
Coconut	*Beef, Venison,*
Dairy[3] (Cheese,	*Pork, etc)*
Cottage Cheese,	**Nuts**
Ice Cream, Milk,	**Olives**
Yogurt	**Seeds**
Eggs	Soybeans
Meat *(Chicken,*	

POOR

FATS & OILS

Avocado Oil	Olive Oil
Butter	*Safflower Oil*
Canola Oil	Green Tea
Coconut Oil	Seed Oil
Corn Oil	*Soy Oil*
Cream	Sesame Oil
Lard	
Nut Oils	

GOOD

CARBOHYDRATES[2]

Beans	Pumpkin
Bread	Split Peas
Brown Rice	Squash *(acorn,*
Cereals	*banana, hub-*
Grains[6]	*bard)*
Lentils	Wheat[6]
Pastas	White Rice
Potatoes	

EXCELLENT

NON-STARCHY VEGETABLES

Asparagus	Eggplant	Radishes
Beet Greens	Endive	Scallions
Broccoli	Escarole	Spinach
Brussels Sprouts	*Garlic*	Sprouts
Cabbage	Green Beans	Summer Squash
Celery	Kale	Sweet Pepper
Chard	Kohlrabi	Swiss Chard
Chicory	Leeks	Tomatoes
Collards	Lettuce	Turnips
Cucumber	Onions	Watercress
Dandelion	Parsley	Zucchini

GOOD · **EXCELLENT** · **EXCELLENT** · **GOOD**

EXCELLENT

MILDLY-STARCHY VEGETABLES

Artichokes	Carrots	Corn
Beets	Cauliflower	Peas

GOOD · **GOOD**

ACID FRUIT

Blackberry	Plum (sour)
Grapefruit	Pomegranate
Lemon/Lime	Raspberry
Orange	Sour Apple
Pineapple	Strawberry

SUB-ACID FRUIT

Apple	Mango
Apricot	Peach
Blueberry	Pear
Cherry	Plum
Kiwi	(sweet)

SWEET FRUIT

Bananas	Papaya
Dates	Persimmon
Currants	Prunes
Figs	Raisins
Grapes	

MELON

Cantaloupe	Watermelon
Casaba	
Crenshaw	
Honeydew	
Persian	

FRUITS are best when eaten **alone**, as a meal, when the stomach is empty of other foods, such as for breakfast. Each fruit group should be eaten separately from other fruit groups, especially melons and sweet fruits.

NOTES

1. ALSO REFER TO ALKALINE/ACID FOODS CHART
2. Carbohydrates and Proteins should never be eaten together, or during the same meal period.
3. Milk and other dairy products are discouraged for human consumption (Exception: mother's breast milk is highly recommended for babies of the same species!)
4. Concentrated proteins are unnecessary. Use as a condiment, not as main course. In any case, eat **no more than** one each meal.
5. Garlic has been reported to produce adverse side effects, and should be considered for medicinal use only.
6. Good when sprouted to vegetable state before consumption.
7. "All things in moderation, including moderation." Socrates
8. This information may be copied and distributed freely.

Probiotics are microorganisms that are friendly to your body. The ones in your digestive system help breakdown some nutrients, such as lactose and gluten and kill paracytes. It is expected that some of the pesticides that you ingest from non-organically grown foods kill your probiotic helpers. There is also evidence that if your digestive system is overly acidic it makes it harder for them to survive and easier for other microorganisms that are not so friendly to survive, such as Candida.

Aside from making sure your digestive system's pH is correct (discusses below), consuming foods with probiotics can help as well. All raw foods have them to some degree, but fermented foods have a higher concentration (ex. dairy/nut yogurts and sauerkrauts).

There are also foods called prebiotics that contain nutrients that help support probiotics. Mainly specific fibers. See *Becoming Super Human* for more information on probiotics, prebiotics[131] and other diet hints.

Acid-Alkaline (pH) is a science of growing importance as we start to recognize that most of us are overly acidic, which makes it difficult for our body to function optimally. The charts on the internet show which food are most acidic forming and which are most alkalizing. Most people need to eat more living foods, such as fruits and vegetables (raw is best) to balance and maintain their pH.

Some people think that taking baking soda will improve their pH. On an completely empty stomach[132] I agree, but before a meal and when a meal is in your stomach, it will only neutralize stomach acids, making it harder on your stomach. Baking soda can also be added to baths, which will often y our skin as it is

---

[131] Prebiotics are foods that support probiotics in our digestive system.

[132] For a completely empty stomach we'll need to wait about 3-4 hours after eating a properly combined meal. Discussed in more depth within *Becoming Super Human*.

absorbed, helping to balance our pH.

Supplements such as multi-vitamins and healthy protein/meal replacement powders are good for people struggling to maintain a health diet. Iodine is of particular importance, because our soils are depleted of it. This is why there are so many people with thyroid problems (iodine is need to make thyroid hormone). Do some research on line to learn more about symptoms of insufficient iodine and how to supplement it. Overdosing on iodine is a big deal, so make sure you know what you are doing!

There are many other supplements that can help us live to our fullest potential. See *Becoming Super Human* and *God's Journey* for more information on supplements and other diet hints.

Cleansing is away of helping our body detoxify, which I discuss in the next Appendix (Appendix E).

Final Comments

To get enough water during the day, you can drink large amount of water when your stomach is empty before meals and sip on water between meals. Try keeping a container of water around at all times to help achieve this.

Getting your heart rate up for 10 minutes a day can make a big difference to your health and performance over time. The increase in blood pressure and circulation helps clean out the smaller areas of your body, improving the blood supply to them. Exercise also helps lymph to circulate in your lymphatic system, which is very important to long term immune system health and performance. A little bit of exercise will get your body craving healthier foods and give you better night sleeps[133]. It is all interconnected!

---

[133] Sufficient sleep is very important to our general health and performance. See *Becoming Super Human* and *God's Journey* for details.

APPENDIX E
LIQUID AND FASTING TYPE CLEANSES

Before getting into these cleanses, know that there are a multitude of cleanses and cleansing products that do not require you to change your diet much. These cleanses are in general less effective, but if your body is heavily toxic, then they are a great start. Such cleanses are increasing the amount of cilantro, italian parsley, garlic, cayenne and other herbs in your diet (see Super-Healthy Beverages in Appendix D for examples). Talking to a health food store and/or exploring information on the internet for other options is a good idea. If wild plants are available, learn what they do and use them. Fresh is always better, especially when they have only been harvested for a few hours.

After a couple of months of eating healthier and/or consuming detoxifying foods and drinks periodically, your body will be ready for a more intensive cleanse that will make noticeable differences to the way you feel, especially during them. Usually people feel enlightened during these cleanses, but if at any time you start to feel nauseous, it could be that you are pushing yourself too hard or not drinking enough water. If this happens, ease off the cleanse, consume more water and slowly return to the cleanse after feeling better.

The cleanses I discuss below help your body shift into a detoxification mode by reducing the activity of the digestive system for an extended period of time. By changing over to a liquid diet, your body works less at digesting and its biochemistry can be devoted to freeing toxins from storage sites and moving them out of your body. Liquid diets are popular, because you can still consume nutrients and energy levels tend to stay the same and even improve. I recommend starting with them.

There are many options for liquid cleanses. In general, they are diets that only consume fresh fruit and vegetable juices made by a juicer. Some modifications of these diets including fresh fruit, lettuces and herbs. I recommend pureeing them first, but these foods are easily digested when chewed sufficiently as well. The herbs play a very important role because they tend to have detoxifying effects that are enhanced when the body is in a detoxification mode. See the Super-Healthy Beverages in Appendix D for examples with cilantro, italian parsley and garlic.

There are special liquid cleanse diets that you can learn more about at health food stores and on the internet. The Master Cleanse is a popular approach with many variations. Essentially it use a combination of alvera juice, lemon juice, a diabetic friendly sweetener and cayenne pepper. This combination fuels the body while minimizing the activity of the digestive system. I have heard of people adding other ingredients to this drink, such as cilantro, italian parsley and garlic; see the internet other modifications.

It is more common to feel a little nauseous during a cleanse when cleansing herbs are used. There are several products that contain herbal formulas to optimize the cleansing experience; the Wild Rose cleanse is a popular example. I recommend drinking a lot of water to avoid this or decreasing the amount of herbs being used. Slowly build up the amount of herbs used. If nausea does occur, ease off the cleansing herbs, keep drinking lots of water, juiced fruits and vegetables[134]. Remember that cilantro needs italian parsley, garlic or chlorophyll rich herb/supplement to be taken with it to help get the metals out of your body. If you do not get enough, it could be the reason for the nausea.

A powerful fruit juice combination is squeezed grapefruit and lemon juice (lots of lemon). This awesome tasting drink has lots of energy and cleansing properties. Be careful not to drink

---

[134] Juiced fruits and vegetables contain lots of antioxidants that will help.

too much or you could get diarrhea. Diarrhea could actually facilitate the cleansing of your intestinal track, because it helps flush solids out. If diarrhea happens, especially if it is intense, you need to make sure you are drinking lots of water, because diarrhea is dehydrating. This cleaning effect is better achieved with colonics hydro therapy or at home enemas; which I recommend and will discussed below.

The next step from a liquid cleanse is to consume nothing but water. I am not sure what cleansing research is saying these days about not consuming anything but water. I imagine there are certain things you can consume that are beneficial for a cleanse like this or have no effect on it. The nothing but water approach has more of an spiritually enlightening effect, which has more of a non-physical cleansing effect than a physical one.

Below I will walk you through a simple liquid cleansing routine

Simple Cleanse Routine

Day 1, going into the cleanse:

Reduce food intake and consume no meat (fish is OK). Increase water intake and do some stretching and light exercise.

Day 2-?[135], in the cleanse:

Do not consume any solid food. Consume only juiced fruits and vegetables, pureed fruits and lettuces, the master cleanse and/or similar beverage and water.

Spend less energy and increase the amount of

---

[135] It is up to we how long we cleanse for. Be mindful of our limits.

time spent in meditation. If you are getting into working with PE, do more of it as well. Spending time in nature is another good idea.

Do this for at least three days and if you feel you can go longer, you should go longer. Some people have done the master cleanse for an entire month. Cleansing for such long periods of time can be the desire to prolong the enlightened feelings that comes with it. Positive emotional states of love and bliss can empower associated PE that make it easier for your body to survive with less nutrients; see *Becoming Super Human* for details. You need to be mindful of your body's limits and patient to experiencing them. The enlightened feelings will come more often and naturally as you progress in this book.

Coming out of the cleanse:

Slowly start introducing solid foods. Try the first day with chopped up fruit and lettuce (not pureed). Start consuming probiotic supplements as well, especially if a parasite cleanse was done (see internet and health food stores for detail on these cleanses).

On the next day, start the same way and then introduce probiotic foods and/or raw and slightly cooked vegetables (sprouts are considered vegetables). Your body will still be in a cleansing mode, so continue to spend less energy, drink adequate water, meditate and practice working with PE.

Start the third day the same way and introduce

well cooked grains and/or beans for lunch. This is the best time to start making healthier choices in your diet and maintaining them, because your digestive system as been partially rest. Your momentum with the cleanse should also make it easier to appreciate the healthier choices and be repelled by the unhealthy ones. This is the time to put in the effort.

In general, cleansing twice a year is a good idea. In the beginning our intuition might guide us to cleanse more often to help make some needed changes.

Colonics and At Home Enemas

Sometimes colon hydrotherapy (aka. Colonics) can greatly facilitate the cleansing process, especially if constipation has been a problem in the past. Hydrotherapy is a machine that flushes your colon with warm water as the practitioner massages your large intestine (aka. colon) walls through your abdomen to help loosen dehydrated food, plaque and other build-ups for the hydrotherapy to take out of your body. Imagine the benefits of removing build ups from your large intestinal walls that produce toxins, house unhealthy parasites and block the absorption of nutrients! Colon toxicity is becoming recognized as a serious source of multiple diseases and disorders.

At Home Enemas are essentially the same thing as colon hydrotherapy, but are harder to do well; see internet and youtube for demos. The hardest thing to duplicate is the flushing motion. I find that exaggerating the expansion and contraction of my abdomen as I breath can serve as a good replacement. The massaging of the practitioner is difficult to do your own as well, but it can be done.

I have found using an electric massaging tool can help improve at home enemas as well as hydrotherapy sessions. The massaging tools vibrations help hydrate build-ups and loosen them in places that the practitioner can not massage easily (ex. transverse section). I recommend these tools for at home enemas and hydrotherapy sessions.

It is truly amazing what this processes has done for people! Consult with an expert and/or do some research on the internet for symptoms that hydrotherapy and enemas can help resolve.

Summary

The idea is to reduce the responsibilities of digestion on the body, so it can focus on detoxification. In the detoxifying state, supplements that promote detoxification will work more effectively. I recommend juicing fruits and vegetables and/or blending fresh herbs that promote detoxification with water or these juices. Lots of local wild plants could work very well for this. If none are available, cilantro, italian parsley and garlic are great herbs that we can get from our grocery store for a low cost (see Super-Healthy Beverage in Appendix D for examples).

Colonics and enemas can greatly help cleanse your body from the other end. Significant health improvements have been observed from these techniques and cleanses in general!

Remember that cleanses can help release unhealthy PE associated with the toxins, cleansing your emotions and mind at the same time. This is one of the big advantages of cleansing for some people. I've seen many people transform from doing a cleanse, especially when combined with a practice involving PE, such as the one discussed in this book.

APPENDIX F
IMPROVING BRAIN HEALTH AND PERFORMANCE

Improving your brain's health and performance makes everything easier, including how well your organs and muscles work. Of central importance, it increases your mental and emotional health and performance. As your brain becomes healthier, mental clarity, problem solving skills, memory, emotional control, emotional stability, intuition and more all increase with it.

Improving your brain's health and performance is basically done the same way as improving your body's, with a few specific differences. In summary, the things that improve your body and brain health and performance are enough water[136], exercise[137] (breathing exercises can supplement physical exercise to a degree), sufficient sleep[138], basic nutrients (vitamins, minerals, protein, carbohydrates and healthy fats)[139], anti-oxidants[140] and detoxification[141].

To make sure you are getting enough of these things, a list can be used to keep track and help you stay diligent. Exercise might tire you out in the beginning, but after you adapt, you'll feel more energized and sleep better, waking up feeling more refreshed.

---

[136] Helps with biochemical reactions and flushing out waste materials.

[137] Increases blood flow, flushing out waste materials from smaller spaces in your body, improving function.

[138] Gives your body a chance to rebuild and reorganize (reorganizing very important for memory formation/learning)

[139] Fuels your body's processes.

[140] Neutralizes free radicals (waste materials), so your body can safely flush them out.

[141] Happens naturally, but many things can help improve this process, making it easier for your body to function.

Sufficient sleep is not always easy. Supplements, brain entrainment and pulsed electromagnetic frequency device can all help get to sleep, sleep deep and wake up. This is a fairly large subject that I discuss in more depth within *Becoming Super Human.*

Getting enough nutrients is not always easy either. Taking a multivitamin with minerals and anti-oxidants can greatly help. I recommend getting these things from fresh foods, but sometime life is too busy to do this well and modern food quality has dropped significantly as well.

Getting enough essential fatty acids (discussed in Appendix D), especially the ones your brain uses a lot of can be difficult from food, because they are rare and easily damaged by processing[142]. There are also more complex brain supplements that work very well. They are in general expensive, but some of them can be very helpful to replace the desire for caffeine[143]!

In Chapter 11 of Dr. Amen's book, *Making a Good Brain Great*, he discusses brain performance diet hints, such as good and bad fat sources, anti-oxidant sources, top twenty-four healthiest brain foods and even gives a grocery store guide to where to find these foods. For more information on advanced brain nutrition for health and performance, see *Becoming Super Human.*

Brain Exercises

Using your brain makes it stronger. Dr. Amen has written a series of books[144] that address similar topics in this book, but from a perspective of increasing physical brain health and performance (no discussion on PE). In Chapter 5 of *Making a*

---

[142] Lots of nutrients are sensitive to processing, such as enzymes. Raw Food diets are the only way to get some nutrients. See Appendix D.

[143] Discussed in more depth within *Becoming Super Human.*

[144] See Amen in references.

Good Brain Great, Dr. Amen gives a brain performance quiz that help identify which of your five major brain regions need improvement and how to improve them with diet, supplements and brain exercises. Very few people have perfect brains, "we all need a little help" [Amen, 2005, p. 70].

Once the brain regions that need enhancement have been identified, you can focus healthy PE upon using similar and the same techniques as discussed in Part 1. An example of this is discussed in the Brain Enhancement Meditation below. This will greatly compliment the more physical approaches.

Focusing PE on your brain is very effective, because your brain is the most interconnected to PE. I have an arm rest shaped like a "T" that positions my hands to rest almost anywhere above my shoulders comfortably (figure 75l). This makes the Brain Enhancement Meditation exercise much easier for long periods of time. Using pillows is another option.

The Brain Enhancement Meditation discusses the nine major brain regions. The better you understand these major brain regions, the better you will be able to hold specific types of PE for them. I discuss this and doing it to the body as well in more detail within *Becoming Super Human* and *Psychic Anatomy Treatments.*

Dr. Amen's books discuss five of the nine major brain regions in regards to enhancing them with nutrients and exercises. Dr. Amen's work, *Becoming Super Human,* as well as other authors[145], can greatly compliment the Brain Enhancement Meditation. New information is always coming out on brain enhancement. I suggest looking for something recent as well.

---

[145]   Part 2 Null, 2005, Mind Power: Rejuvenating Your Brain and Memory Naturally, and Amen, 2008, Magnificent Mind at Any Age: Natural Ways to Unleash Your Brain's Maximum Potential,for other approaches with many ideas on specific brain conditions.

Remember, your brain is extremely important to living to your fullest potential!

Brain Enhancement Meditation

You have the option of doing some Psychic Anatomy Yoga help charge yourself up with healthy PE before doing this exercise. When you are ready, get comfortable, relax and release yourself into a meditative state lying down (a good time is before going to bed[146]). Focus on breathing, as you make your way to holding your palms towards your physical heart (figure 75a), holding healthy PE there. This will help tune your entire physical body to healthy PE[147].

When you are ready, move your palms to your forehead or just above it (figure 75b), holding healthy PE on your Frontal Lobes[148]. Visualize your frontal lobes glowing to help focus PE there (use this visualization for each brain region below). When you feel like you have done enough, move your hands to place your palms slightly behind your temples, fingers above your ears to hold healthy PE at your Temporal Lobes (figure 75c). When you feel you have spent enough time here, move to your Parietal Lobes (figure 75d), followed by your Visual Lobes (figure 75e), Cingulate Gyrus (figure

---

[146] Use pillows and/or blankets to help hold your arms up if necessary.
[147] Heartmath has done a lot of research with the heart in regards to this tuning.
[148] Your prefrontal lobes are the most important part of your frontal lobes.

75f), Limbic System[149] (figure 75g), Thalamus (figure 75h), Brain Stem (figure 75i) and then Cerebellum (figure 75j). Finish at your heart (figure 75k), focusing on balancing and harmonizing your brain, body and heart.

Figure 75l shows the posture for charging your limbic system using a Meditation T. These Meditation Ts make it much more comfortable to do this exercise sitting up. I highly recommend Meditation Ts to help get in the habit of charging your brain more often (your brain is extremely important for living to your fullest potential). A large pillow can be used as well, but it doesn't work as well as a Meditation T. They are very easy to make. See Appendix H.

Example Affirmation

"I am enhancing the health and performance of my frontal lobes". Repeat for each brain region with their name in replace of frontal lobes.

---

[149] Made up of several regions.

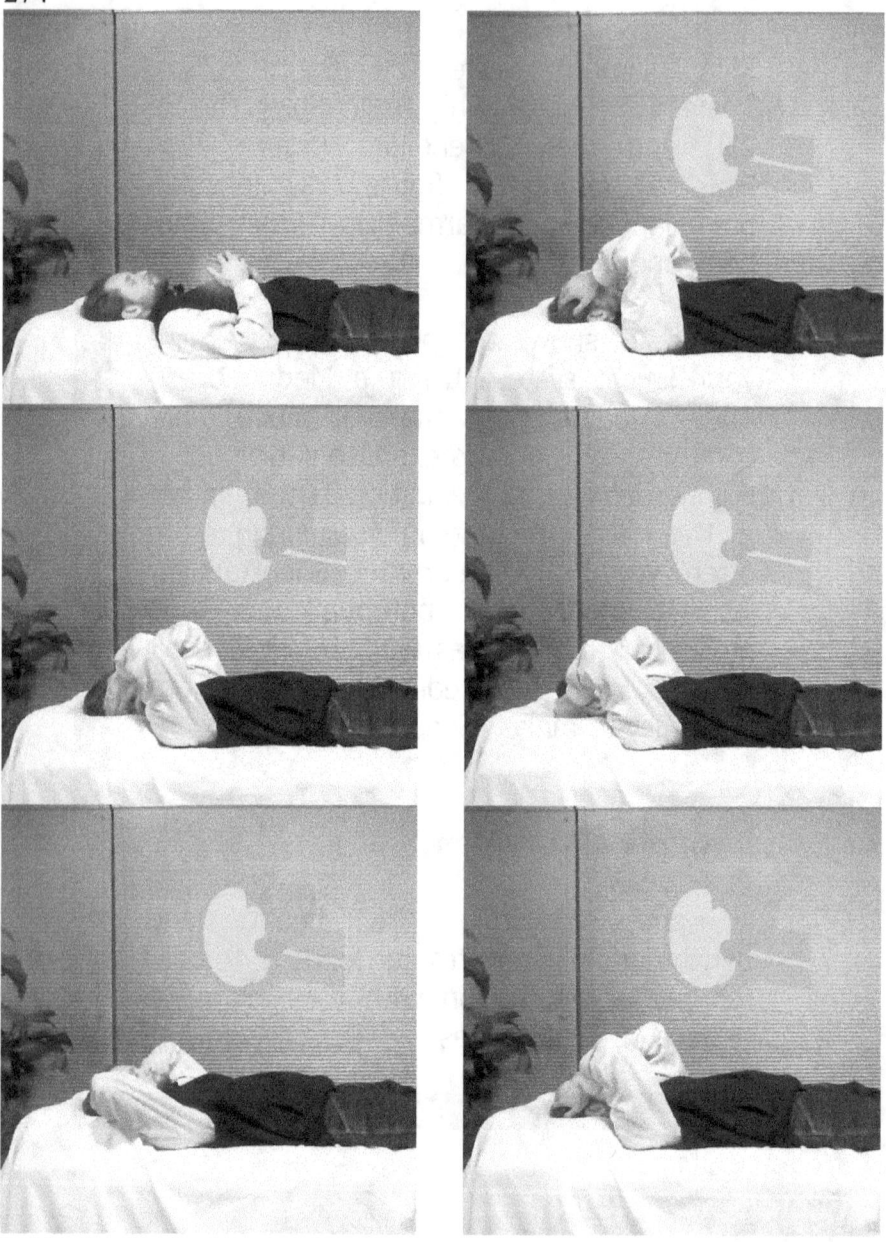

Figure 75a-f: Top Left (a), tuning body to healthy PE using the physical heart. Top right (b), charging of frontal lobes. Middle left (c), charging of temporal lobes. Middle right (d), charging of parietal lobes. Bottom left (e), charging of visual lobes. Bottom right (f), charging of cingulate gyrus.

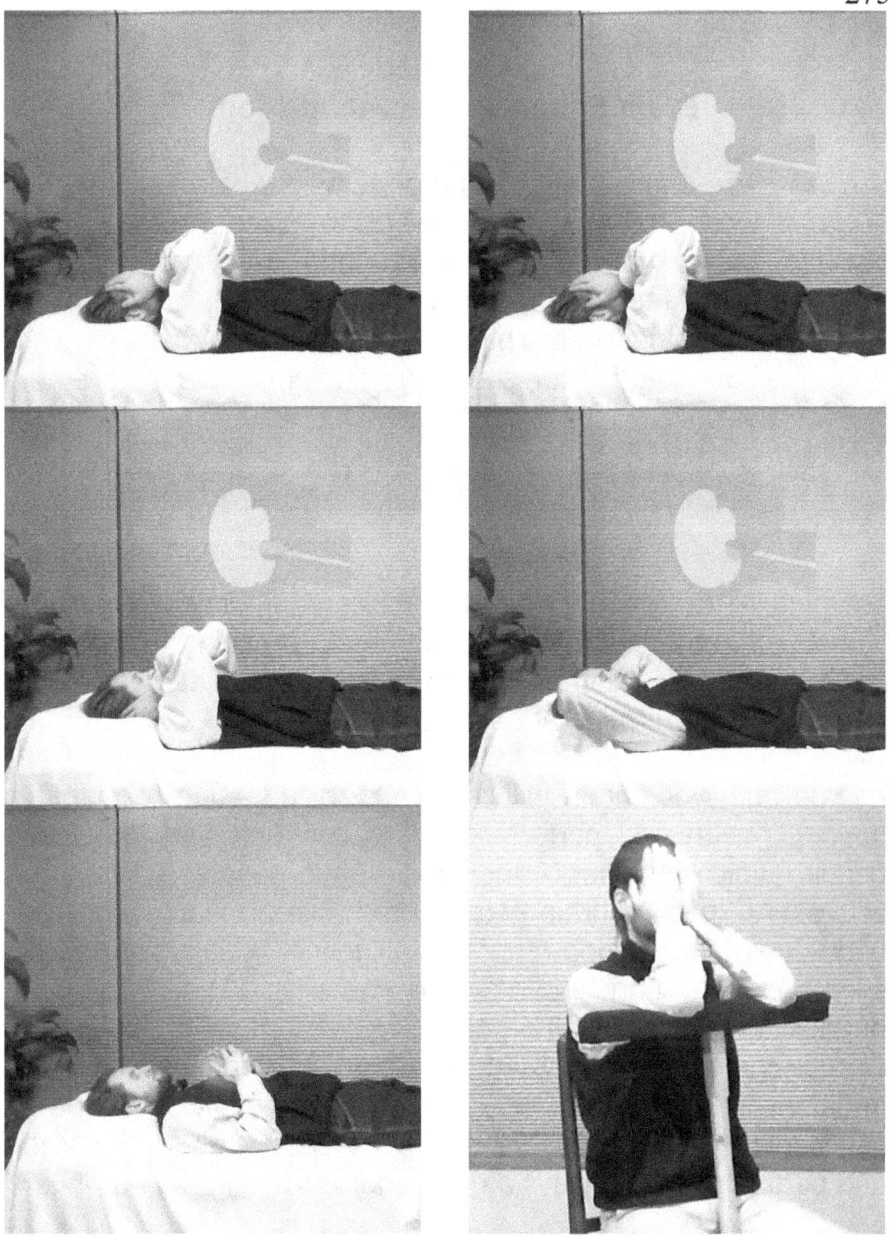

Figure 75g-l: Top left (g), charging of limbic system. Top right (h), charging of thalamus. Middle left (i), charging of brain stem. Middle right (j), charging of cerebellum. Bottom right (k), reinforcing tuning body to healthy PE using the physical heart. Bottom right (l), example of using Meditation T.

Simplified
Brain Enhancement Meditation

The entire brain can be done as a whole as well.   Ultimately you want to place your hands where it feels right (intuitively), but such feelings will not always exist.   I recommend the hands position in figures 75f, g and h for charging your entire brain at once.

Learning to do anything new exercises your brain. The more complex it is the better. Decreasing brain numbing things, such as TV, some video games and drugs also helps keep your brain healthy and performing at its best.

As you age, your brain will require extra attention to maintain optimal health and performance. A common one for elderly people, which is opposite for middle aged people, is keeping it active. An inactive brain gets sluggish like an inactive physical body does. To develop mental intelligence, you simply need to stimulate it.   Enriching reading material, doing crossword puzzles and other mind-games[150], engaging in intellectual discussions, doing visualizations, doing affirmations and using intuition are good examples. Learning something new that is applicable to your purpose and/or mind-body-spirit (MBS) health and performance is always a good choice as well.

---

[150]   Search free "mind/brain games" online.

Learning gets easier the more you do it, its like a muscle.

Some people overuse their brains and actually need to give it a break, allowing it to rejuvenate. Mindless tasks do this and allow for intuition and reflection to get your attention more easily. Working in a garden, spending time in nature, cleaning, the Spontaneous Expression Exercises discussed in Chapter 4 of *Inner and Outer Success* and simple meditative practices, such as just focusing on your breath for long periods of time are good brain rejuvenation techniques.

An over worked brain can be prevented and recovered from more easily with supplements and techniques. I discuss this in depth within *Becoming Super Human.*

Avoiding diet choices that harm the brain is of course a good choice as well. "As little caffeine as possible is a good rule, if you want to respect and nurture your brain" [Amen, 2005, p. 83]. You need to save caffeine and other stimulants for when you really need them, such as making a deadline or driving. Is it really necessary to be fully alert when watching TV, relaxing or socializing? Getting comfortable with being in a rejuvenation mode helps you sleep and relax more, improving your health and performance. There is a lot you can do with low energy, basically anything you find easy. Charging yourselves with healthy PE is a great example that will also speed up the process of rejuvenation.

Brain Hemisphere Balancing

Your left and right brain hemispheres work differently, and they need to work together for optimal brain performance. These hemispheres can go out of sync with one dominating your mental perspective if it is overused. There are various things you can do to help balance them and keep them balanced. This can bring about a much more centered perspective and optimized brain performance.

There are a few programs that help balance brain hemispheres using exercises, such as Brain Gym and the Brain Balance Program. Bilateral beats are my favorite, which are easier to use, but less specific. They use two slightly different sound frequencies that require your two hemispheres to work together to make sense of the sound. It has been shown to balance brain hemispheres very well. They can also induce brain states associated with different states of alertness, such as sleep, meditation (relaxed state), causal-alertness and hyper-alertness[151].

The Brain Enhancement Meditation and the Simplified Brain Enhancement Meditation can include intentions of balancing left and right sides of each brain region and the whole brain as well.

Summary

No matter what you are trying to do in your life, improving your brain's health and performance will make it easier.

---

[151] Search "bilateral beat research" online and/or see *Becoming Super Human*.

APPENDIX G
THE EIGHT LIMBS OF
PSYCHIC ANATOMY YOGA

**The Eight Limbs of
Psychic Anatomy Yoga**

Yamas: Control of behavior to fit a virtuous code.

Niyamas: Control of perspective to fit a virtuous code.

Asanas: Control of the body to challenge the mind, promote physical health and performance as well as the health and performance of the koshas (sheaths/psychic anatomy).

Pranayama: Control of breath and life force (prana).

Pratyahara: With drawl from the physical senses, which includes the emotions and thoughts birthed by the brain/ego[152]. Emotional and/or mental awareness of PE is good; see Dharana.

Dharana: Becoming attuned to your awareness as a result of achieving Pratyahara.

---

[152] Most desires are based by brain processes/ego. Pratyahara is a serious art.

Dhyana: To devote Dharana to enlightenment. Connecting to higher states of consciousness. Ultimately connecting to God.

Samadhi: Union with higher states of consciousness. Ultimately union with God.

Psychic Anatomy Yoga aids greatly in the purpose of the asanas. It challenges the mind more with added tasks, promotes physical health and performance better because of the mind-body-spirit connection and more directly facilitates the health and performance of the koshas (aka. psychic anatomy).

The more physically parts of your psychic anatomy work with life force/prana, such as your meridians and internal aura. Although it is not taught in the depth within this book that it is in Level 5 of *The Psychic Anatomy Exercises,* control of life force/prana (pranayama) can be an important part of Psychic Anatomy Yoga practice.

Pratyahara and Dharana are developed as a consequence of becoming more aware of PE, which Psychic Anatomy Yoga helps develop. By working with and enhancing the health and performance of your psychic anatomy, you become more consciously aware of it as well as PE. Your awareness of PE comes from your psychic anatomy.

Dhyana is a choice that I recommend you devote your practice to. As you become more enlightened, you will become aware of specific devotions that compliment your purpose in life. For example, connecting to states of consciousness that make you a better parent, teacher and/or leader etc.

Practicing Psychic Anatomy Yoga accelerates progress with Dhyana by helping to Descend the associated PE to be embodied by your physical body (ex. DNA and other biocrystals[153]). Many people will reach great states of enlightenment briefly, but to embody/resonant with these PE all the time, takes practice.

Some people hardly eat (fast) for long periods of time to make it easier to stay connected to these states of consciousness as they learn to embody them. This can have several consequences to their physical health and especially physical performance. Psychic Anatomy Yoga uses the science of psychic anatomy and the process of embodying higher states of consciousness to facilitate the process. See *The Psychic Anatomy Exercises* and *Psychic Anatomy Treatments* for more information on the concepts and exercises for greatly enhancing this embodiment process.

Samadhi is achieving a state of union with (embodying the PE of) higher states of consciousness/God. You can also form samadhi with aspects of consciousness that help you become a better parent, teacher and/or leader, etc. Ultimately, union with God takes a path through your higher states of consciousness, which will guide you to embody aspects of consciousness to live to your fullest potential as a part of creation's/God's evolution. See *God's Journey* for more on this perspective.

---

[153] Discussed in more depth within *The Interface Between Psychic Energies and the Physical Body.*

APPENDIX H

MAKING A KNEELING STOOL, MEDITATION T AND WRIST/ANKLE SUPPORT BLOCKS

Many people will find these very easy to make. For those who do not have the tools, skills and/or want a fancy made Kneeling Stool, Meditation T and/or Wrist/Ankle Support Block, you will eventually be able to order one from us.

Making a Kneeling Stool

You will need for the Kneeling Stool:
- 3 feet of 2x6 lumber
- Saw
- Measuring tape or ruler
- 4 #8x3 inch wood screws
- Drill and 1/8 drill bit (optional)
- Wood glue (optional)
- 4 corner brackets (optional)

You will need for foam cushion:
- A 12x6 inch piece of foam; you choose thickness.
- Another 12x6 inch piece of foam; you choose thickness. (optional)
- Enough fabric to cover foam. You can also use duct tape ;) .
- Staple gun or carpet tacks

On your 30 inch piece of 2x6, mark on the edge, 5 inches from each end length-wise. On the other edge, mark 6 inches from the length-wise end to make the Kneeling Stool Legs (see figure 76). Cut a line between the 5 inch and 6 inch marks. Straighten the ends of your remaining piece, which should be about 18 inches for your Kneeling Stool's seat (figure 77).

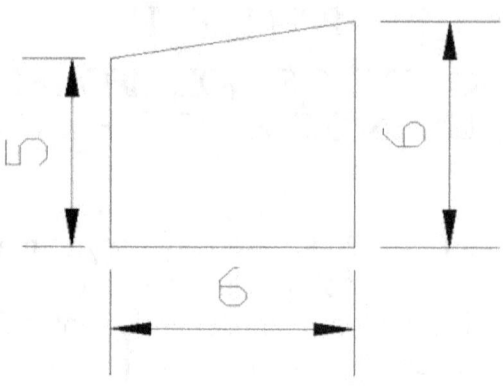

Figure 76: Side view of Kneeling Stool Leg.

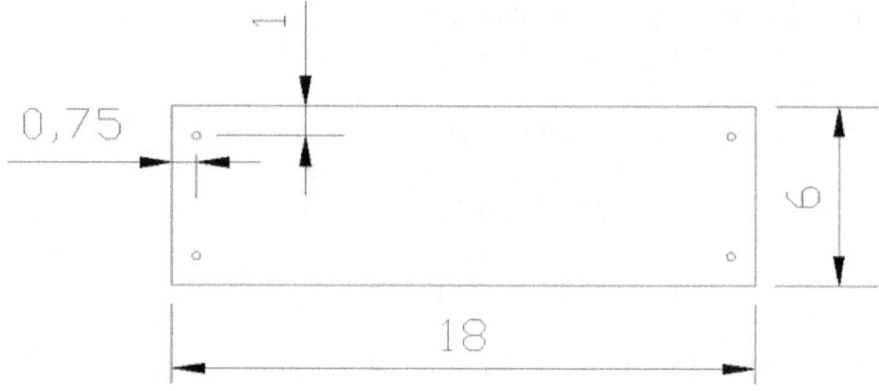

Figure 77: Top view of Kneeling Stool Seat. Circle are the guide holes.

Drill some guide hole for the screws, this will insure the wood does not crack when putting in the screws. First mark out the holes as shown in figure 77. Press in with a screw to make an indent to help guide the 1/8 drill bit. Be mindful of drilling into your table ;). Next, place the seat on the legs and hold one end aligned as you drill two wholes into the leg threw the holes in the seat. Next, remove the seat and drill deeper into the legs. Now do the other side.

Putting some wood glue between the legs and seat before screwing them together will make their connection stronger. You can also instal some corner brackets to make it even stronger. They are not needed if you are careful not to put too much weight on the legs when using the Kneeling Stool as a support block. Put all your weight on the seat part and install the screws.

Now you have a Kneeling Stool.

If you want to instal cushions, put one piece of foam on top (and one on the bottom; optional) and wrap your piece of fabric around to make sure it is long and wide enough. You need to have about twice the width to make sure the fabric is wide enough to fold under the foam for a clean finish. The cushion underneath is intended for using the Kneeling Stool as a pillow.

Assuming you have enough length, fold about 1/2 inch of the length-end of fabric and staple the center of it to the back-center of the seat (narrow part of seat above the higher end of legs). Work your way to the edges of the foam, folding the fabric under the foam width-edges to create a clean edge once you complete stapling. Fold the fabric around the top piece of foam (and bottom piece if you include it), folding the width-edges under the same way and staple the other length-end of the fabric to have approximately a 1/2 inch folded under again to the back of the seat again (overlapping the first set of staples).

You can also just use duct tape or another tape to cover the foam. If you do this, wrap the foam in a plastic bag to protect it in case you want to remove the tape in the future. I don't recommend this approach, but it is a lot easier.

Making Meditation T

You'll need for the Meditation T:
- 15-24 inch piece of 2x2
- Probably a saw
- 24 inch piece of 1x4
- 2 corner brackets
- 4 #6x1/2 inch screws

You'll need for foam cushion:
- 1x4 piece of foam (you choose thickness)
- Fabric, duct tape or socks
- Staple gun or carpet tacks

Sitting in a chair with a straight spine, measure the distance from the chair seat to your nipple. This is the approximate perfect length for the 2x2. If you cut it longer you can always cut it shorter later on.

Mount the 2x2 piece to the center of the 1x4 with the corner brackets. No guide holes are needed. You now have a Meditation T.

To add a foam cushion, make sure you have enough fabric to cover the foam piece. Start by folding over one end of the fabric about a 1/2 inch. Staple its center close to the center of the 1x4's length on the bottom side. Work your way to the ends. Do the same on the other side. You may need to fold over more or less than 1/2inch to make a clean edge. You should have some flaps at the ends that you can fold up and staple under the 1x4 for a clean finish.

You can also just duct tape the foam to the 1x4. If you do so, I recommend wrapping the foam in plastic bags so you can remove the tape later on without damaging the foam.

You can also just use soaks (no foam).

Making Wrist/Ankle Support Blocks

You'll need to make Wrist/Ankle Support Blocks:
- 2 12x6 inch pieces of 3/8 plywood or thicker
- A file, rough sandpaper or an adjustable saw

Take your 12x6 inch pieces of plywood and create a slope on all of its sides using a file, sandpaper or a saw (figure 78). Figure shows a 45-degree slope. You'll have to find the angles that work best for you. Try a different angle on each end. You may also want to shorten/lengthen one side so it fits better in your hand/foot. In the future I might carry these blocks made of rubber for a better fit and stick.

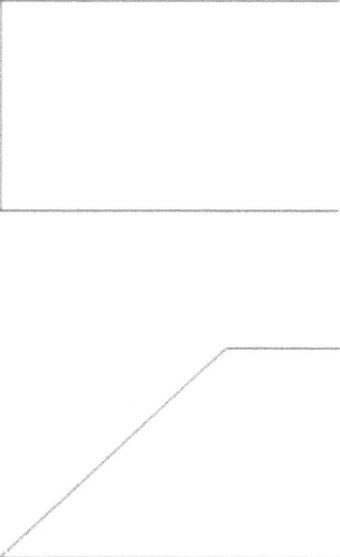

Figure 78: Side view of Wrist/Ankle Support Blocks. Top view is before creating the slope. Bottom view is after creating the slope.

About the Author

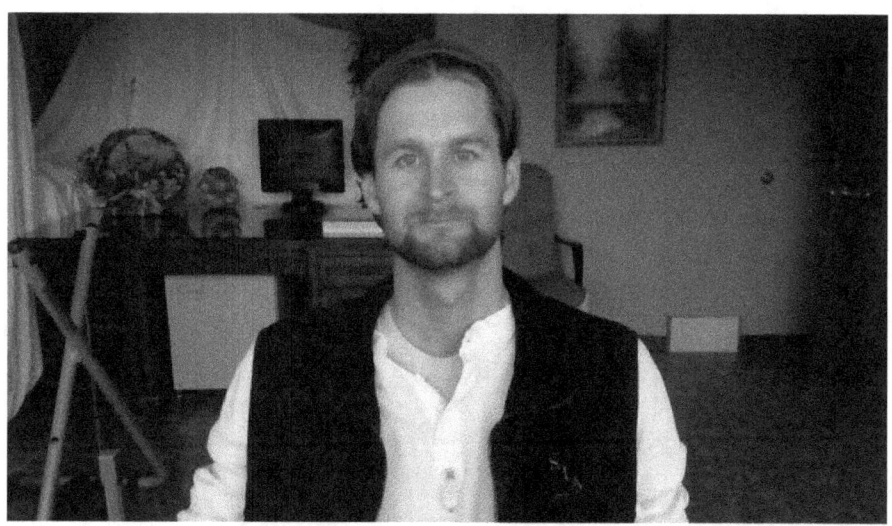

Brett A. Rogers has always been passionate about the meaning of life. Since about 1997 he has recognized that learning and improving upon the psychological and physical foundations we are built upon, makes it easier to identify and express the meaning of life. He has pursued enlightenment of these subjects in the formal and informal academic study of physics, neuroscience, psychology, physiology, nutrition, metaphysics and spirituality. Metaphysics and spirituality are not considered pure academic sciences yet, but Brett has been very diligent in collecting and communicating academically relevant information concerning these subjects to help develop them as a science.

In 1995, Brett A. Rogers was introduced to meditation and Energy Healing-Empowerment by his mother. They exchanged many Energy Healing-Empowerment treatments (reiki) for many years, giving him many benefits[154]. When he entered university in 1998, he started to study and practice metaphysics and spiritually as a science along with his university classes. He

---

[154] Brett emphasizes the importance of receiving regular Energy Healing-Empowerment treatments for optimal health and performance (weekly).

spent 7 years of formal and informal study at the University of Saskatchewan.

Once leaving the academic world, his life provided great freedoms for him to continue his studies and practices. In 2006, he started to write his first books, The Psychic Energy Reality and The Psychic Anatomy Exercises. With a diligent practice, which included many practices that involved psychic energies (aka. chi, prana, ki, emotional and mental energies, the energies of our psyche) (ex. Energy Healing-Empowerment, meditation, Psychic Anatomy Exercises and more), he continued to study and write for several years until feeling guided to start to publishing his work in 2012 (see the following pages for an introduction to some of his other books).

From instructional media on how to enhance our health and performance using conventional and psychic energy techniques, to opinions about priorities of personal and collective evolution, Brett A. Rogers covers a large ground of subjects and ties them all together as significant to personal and collective evolution. His used of simple English and underlining passion makes all of his books an easy and inspiring read.

Learn more about Brett A. Rogers at his website: www.ourevolution.co.nr

OTHER BOOKS & DVDS
BY BRETT A. ROGERS

MORE INFORMATION ON THESE BOOKS &
DVDS CAN BE FOUND @

WWW.OUREVOLUTION.CO.NR

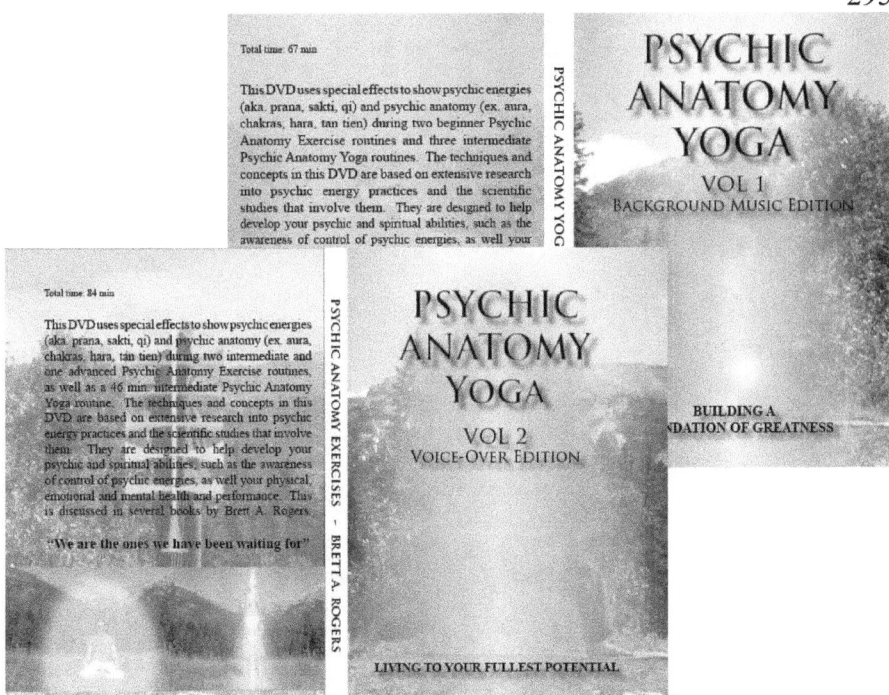

Total time: 67 min

This DVD uses special effects to show psychic energies (aka. prana, sakti, qi) and psychic anatomy (ex. aura, chakras, hara, tan tien) during two beginner Psychic Anatomy Exercise routines and three intermediate Psychic Anatomy Yoga routines. The techniques and concepts in this DVD are based on extensive research into psychic energy practices and the scientific studies that involve them. They are designed to help develop your psychic and spiritual abilities, such as the awareness of control of psychic energies, as well your

PSYCHIC ANATOMY YOGA

PSYCHIC ANATOMY YOGA
VOL 1
BACKGROUND MUSIC EDITION

BUILDING A FOUNDATION OF GREATNESS

Total time: 84 min

This DVD uses special effects to show psychic energies (aka. prana, sakti, qi) and psychic anatomy (ex. aura, chakras, hara, tan tien) during two intermediate and one advanced Psychic Anatomy Exercise routines, as well as a 46 min. intermediate Psychic Anatomy Yoga routine. The techniques and concepts in this DVD are based on extensive research into psychic energy practices and the scientific studies that involve them. They are designed to help develop your psychic and spiritual abilities, such as the awareness of control of psychic energies, as well your physical, emotional and mental health and performance. This is discussed in several books by Brett A. Rogers.

"We are the ones we have been waiting for"

PSYCHIC ANATOMY EXERCISES — BRETT A. ROGERS

PSYCHIC ANATOMY YOGA

PSYCHIC ANATOMY YOGA
VOL 2
VOICE-OVER EDITION

LIVING TO YOUR FULLEST POTENTIAL

DVDs

These DVDs used special effects to show psychic energies and psychic anatomy during Psychic Anatomy Exercises, Psychic Anatomy Yoga and Psychic Anatomy Treatment routines. With stunning backgrounds, these routines are presented with voice over to help communicate the concepts. They are a great compliments to the books for learning, as well as motivating you to practice more often and for longer periods of time.

Brett presents seminars and teaches workshops/classes on some of the information discussed in this book.

See www.ourevolution.co.nr for more information and ordering

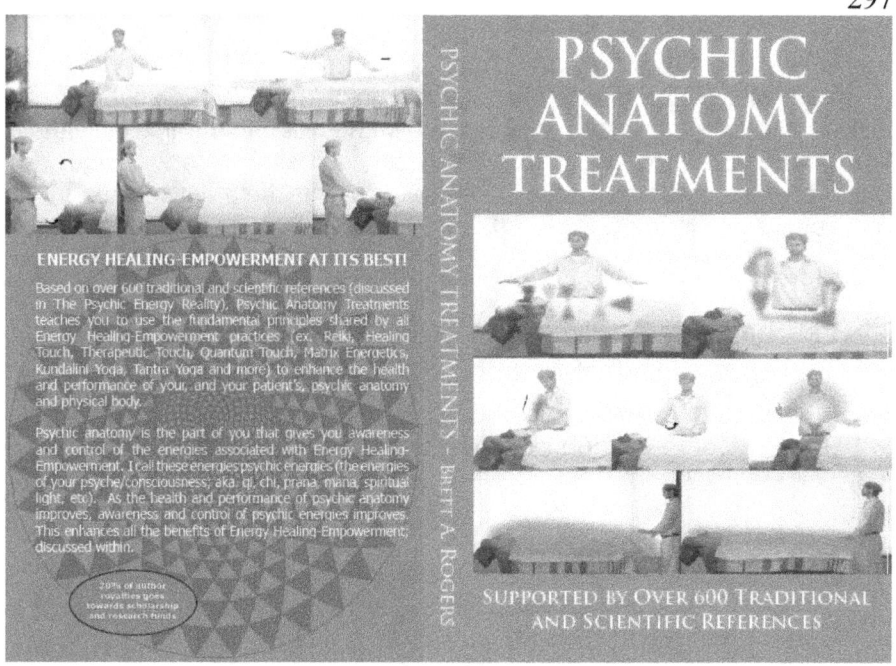

PSYCHIC ANATOMY TREATMENTS
ENERGY HEALING-EMPOWERMENT AT ITS BEST!:
SUPPORTED BY OVER 600 TRADITIONAL AND
SCIENTIFIC REFERENCES

Based on over 600 supporting traditional and scientific references (discussed in *The Psychic Energy Reality*), Psychic Anatomy Treatments teaches you how to use the fundamental principles shared by all Energy Healing-Empowerment practices (ex. Reiki, Quantum Touch, Matrix Energetics, BodyTalk, Kundalini Yoga and more) to enhance the health and performance of the psychic anatomy and physical body of the person you are treating, as well as your own.

As your psychic anatomy improves, your abilities to both consciously and unconsciously utilize and work with the energies associated with it, which I call psychic energies (the energies of our psyche/consciousness; aka. qi, prana, mana, life force, bioenergy, etc), improves as well. This gives you, and the people you treat, faster and more noticeable results from all Energy Healing-Empowerment practices, as well as related practices. Of particular importance is improved intuition, as well as improved awareness and power with psychic energies.

Psychic anatomy is the part of you that serves as the bridge between your human-self and higher aspects of your consciousness, this is why enhancing its health and performance enhances your intuition. Psychic anatomy also acts as the interface between the psychic energies around you and those within you. Learning to enhance the health and performance of your and other people's psychic anatomy, will give you and them advantages in life that you may never have expected.

Brett presents seminars and teaches workshops/classes on some of the information discussed in this book.

See www.ourevolution.co.nr for more information and ordering

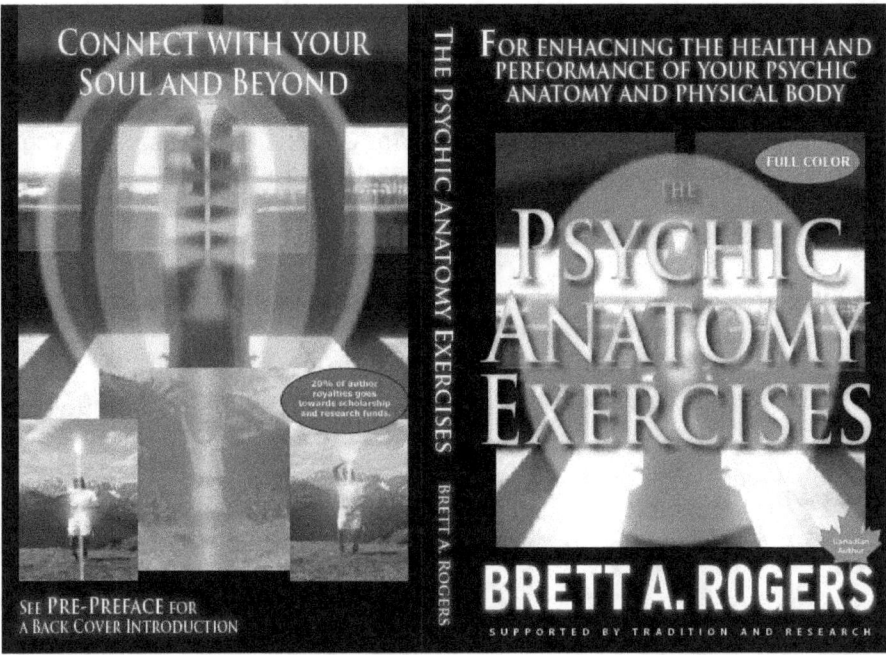

THE PSYCHIC ANATOMY EXERCISES

FOR ENHANCING THE HEALTH AND PERFORMANCE OF YOUR PSYCHIC ANATOMY AND PHYSICAL BODY:

SUPPORTED BY TRADITION AND RESEARCH

The Psychic Anatomy Exercises are a set of meditative exercises that empower the health and performance of your psychic anatomy (ex. chakras, aura, meridians, nadis, tan tien, hara and more). This enhances your emotional, mental and of course psychic health and performance, giving you greater awareness and control of yourself and the psychic energies around you. Intuition is a special type of psychic energy awareness that has tremendous advantages to the decision rich lifestyles many of you lead, especially in the areas of business and sports. Being more aware of your intuitive feelings helps you sense when something will or will not work before investing time and energy into trying.

Our psychic anatomy interfaces with your physical body in many ways. This is the mind-body-spirit connection. As the health and performance of your psychic anatomy increases or decreases, your body reflects this. Psychic Anatomy Exercises enhances your physical health and performance by reducing the presence of unhealthy psychic energies within you and empowering the healthier ones.

The Psychic Anatomy Exercises can be considered a modernized version of Qigong, Energy Healing-Empowerment, Tai Chi and some forms of Yoga. These changes are the result of the research and experiences of Brett A. Rogers; discussed in *The Psychic Energy Reality.*

Brett presents seminars and teaches workshops/classes on the information discussed in this book.

See www.ourevolution.co.nr for more information and ordering.

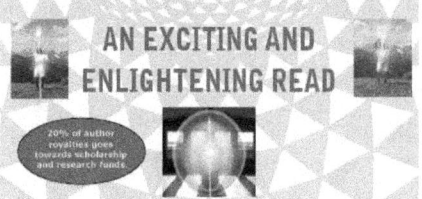

THE PSYCHIC ENERGY REALITY
A TRADITIONAL AND ACADEMIC FOUNDATION FOR PSYCHIC ENERGY PRACTICES AND RESEARCH: OVER 600 SUPPORTING REFERENCES

The Psychic Energy Reality is an important book for those seeking truth about reality, spiritual enlightenment, psychic abilities and more. It discusses topics familiar with most people and expands upon them using traditional and scientific references to support the ideas discussed. An amazing read for first time explorers of psychic and spiritual concepts, a must for all who engage in a psychic or spiritual practice! The information on psychic anatomy will inspire you and the references convince you that they are real and important to your and your evolution.

Brett A. Rogers has studied and practiced in these fields since 1995 and has developed a psychic energy practice called Psychic Anatomy Exercises that utilize the information in this book.

Brett presents seminars and teaches workshops/classes on the information discussed in this book.

See www.ourevolution.co.nr for more information and ordering.

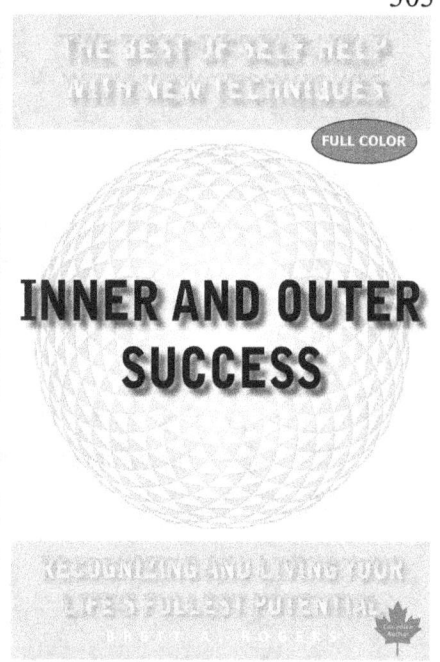

INNER AND OUTER SUCCESS
THE BEST OF SELF-HELP WITH NEW TECHNIQUES:
RECOGNIZING AND LIVING YOUR
LIFE'S FULLEST POTENTIAL

Inner and Outer Success is a self-help book that teaches the best of conventional self-help techniques while incorporating meditative techniques and Psychic Anatomy Exercises. The meditative techniques and Psychic Anatomy Exercises help empower healthy psychic energies within you, which causes a detox of unhealthy psychic energies associated with your inner issues (ex. unhealthy emotions and thoughts). This book focuses on empowering you in several ways that causes the healing (neutralizing) of inner issues to happen spontaneously and often effortlessly. This and related psychic energy phenomenon are being explored in several sub-fields of psychology and medicine.

Techniques for self-exploration, improving self-awareness, living simply, managing relationships, managing yourselves and enhancing your physical health are also discussed in regards to conventional self-help techniques and psychic energies. The potential of psychic energies to enhance your health and performance has been known since the beginning of recorded time, but only recently has it been met with academic research, resulting in incredible advancements on how you can used them.

Brett A. Rogers has been diligently studying and practicing psychic energy arts since 1995. He has written several books on these subjects, which have contributed to the information presented in this one.

Brett presents seminars and teaches workshops/classes on some of the information discussed in this book.

See www.ourevolution.co.nr for more information and ordering

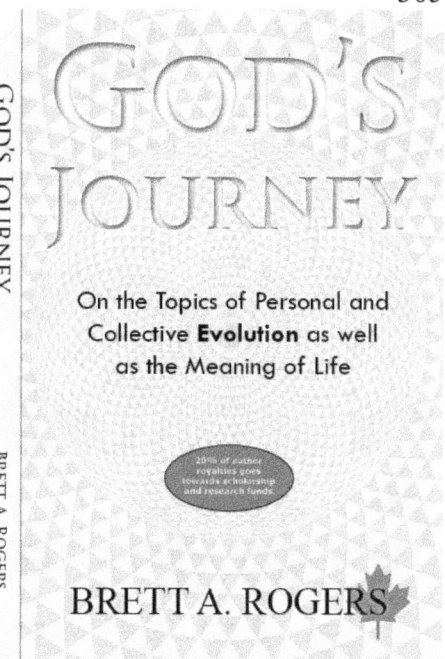

GOD'S JOURNEY
ON THE TOPICS OF PERSONAL AND COLLECTIVE EVOLUTION, AS WELL AS THE MEANING OF LIFE

God's Journey is probably the most important book Brett A. Rogers has written so far. It discusses the topics of personal and collective evolution, as well as provides steps to help you move in these directions. Many topics are just introduced with references and guidance for learning more provided, while others are discussed in more depth. The topics surrounding emotional and mental energies are revisited several times as important factors to optimizing your personal and collective evolution while other topics are being and independently. His statements regarding these energies are an eye opener to the importance of this part of reality that many of you are only partially aware of.

His comments are logical and religiously neutral. He does however discuss a perspective of reality that is commonly agreed upon by spiritually minded people. This perspective is not needed for his guidance on optimizing your personal and collective evolution, but it does set a simple foundation for his perspective on the Meaning of Life.

THIS BOOK IS NOT YET PUBLISHED

BECOMING SUPER HUMAN

With the recent and rapid advances of your science and technology, becoming super human is a now reality. Becoming Super Human focuses on the subjects of advanced nutrition, psychic energy practices and the used of natural and artificial electromagnetic rhythms to enhance the health and performance of your physical body and psychic anatomy. These topics many sound complicated, but Mr. Rogers does an excellent job at presenting them with simplicity, using boxed off information and references to take the reader deeper when they choose. He even presents a simple and inexpensive design that he useds exclusively to empower himself with electromagnetic rhythms.

With the information in this book and some motivation, anyone can develop a comprehension of the information within it and used it to make significant improvements to their immediate and future health and performance. Its much easier than you may think and its all here in one book!

Brett presents seminars and teaches workshops/classes on some of the information discussed in this book.

THIS BOOK IS NOT YET PUBLISHED

THE INTERFACE BETWEEN PSYCHIC ENERGIES AND THE PHYSICAL BODY

The Interface Between Psychic Energies and the Physical Body discusses how the physical body useds electromagnetic waves in its physical design and as an interface with psychic energies and psychic anatomy. Of particular importance is its sensitivity to low intensities that match those observed in association with psychic energies. These observations and associated theories are written for everybody in a clear and precise way with lots of in depth information being boxed off.

This interface has been identified in bits and pieces for a number of years, but no one has done a comprehensive review of the observations and tied them all together as presented in this book. Doing so has resulted in great insights into the questions of human consciousness, how the brain works, emotional and mental contagion, psychosomatics and more. Of particular importance is how these insights can be applied to technology. Technologies that used electromagnetic rhythms to enhance the health and performance of living creatures already exist (a simple and inexpensiv e design is presented within). These technologies are reviewed with comments on innovating them, as well as future research directions.

This book is leading edge!

Brett presents seminars and teaches workshops/classes on some of the information discussed in this book.

THIS BOOK NOT YET PUBLISHED

THE NEW MILITARY

The New Military is a series of fictional stories that start with a story about a Military General who lost his son to a plane bombing that he could have avoided by trusting his intuition. When forced to search through old research materials that he and his son worked on together, his memories of this past trauma trigger an awakening of his psychic gifts. With some help from his daughter and her boy friend, this awakening is accelerated in the environment of an observing and concerned family, coworkers and a visiting Corporal General over viewing a project that his intuition warns him of potential danger.

Proceeding books tell the story of how a military starts to train soldiers to develop their psychic abilities and the used of technology to amplify some of these abilities to stop wars and create resolution. These books are filled with guidance, knowledge, humor, powerful messages and the potential for an incredible series of movies.

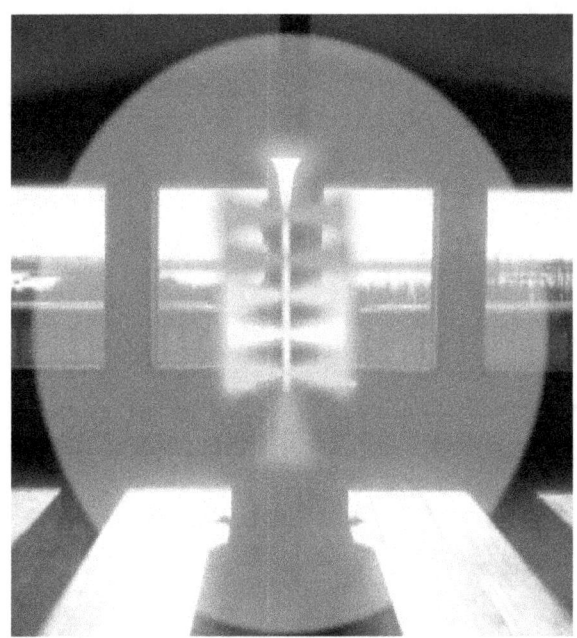

In Person and Online Events

Retreats, workshops, classes and seminars can be participated in person and online, giving you the opportunity to ask questions in the moment, be guided directly on using various techniques, facilitated in many ways, experience the fantastic energies cultivated, meet and socialize with like minded people and much more.

I (Brett A. rogers) work closely with Angels, Ascended Masters (aka. the souls of the spiritually adept), gemstones, sacred geometry and sacred sound to co-create an incredible healing and empowering experience for all events. This is usually more profound during in person events, although learning to work with angels, ascended masters and fields of collective consciousness can make it easier to empower these experiences from a far. How to do this is discussed in a few of my books, as well as most of the in person and online events.

Guided Meditations and Mini-Energy Healing-Empowerment treatments are included with most events; in person and online.

:) Please visit www.ourevolution.co.nr for more information :)